Understanding Herpes

Understanding Health and Sickness Series
Miriam Bloom, Ph.D.
General Editor

Understanding Herpes

Revised Second Edition

Lawrence R. Stanberry, M.D., Ph.D.

University Press of Mississippi
Jackson

www.upress.state.ms.us

The University Press of Mississippi is a member of
the Association of American University Presses.

Copyright © 2006 by University Press of Mississippi
All rights reserved
Manufactured in the United States of America

Illustrations by Regan Causey Tuder
Originally published in 1998
Revised second edition 2006

Library of Congress Cataloging-in-Publication Data

Stanberry, Lawrence R.
    Understanding herpes / Lawrence R. Stanberry.
        p. cm. — (Understanding health and sickness series)
    Includes index.
    ISBN 1-57806-867-3 (cloth : alk. paper) — ISBN 1-57806-868-1
(pbk. : alk. paper) 1. Herpes genitalis. 2. Herpes simplex. I. Title.
II. Understanding health and sickness series.
    RC203.H45 S73   2006
    616.95'18—dc22   2005054690

British Library Cataloging-in-Publication Data available

Contents

Acknowledgments

I dedicate this second edition of *Understanding Herpes* to the memory of my friend and longtime colleague, Stephen Sacks, M.D., an internationally recognized genital herpes expert—he was both an exceptional clinical researcher and a tireless patient advocate. Steve died in November 2003 after a lengthy illness; he is much missed.

This second edition contains new information regarding the diagnosis and treatment of genital herpes, including breakthrough new discoveries about how three-, two-, and even one-day courses of antiviral therapy can be effective in the treatment of herpes outbreaks. A section has been added that discusses frightening new data about how genital herpes appears to increase the risk of acquiring and transmitting human immunodeficiency virus (HIV), the cause of acquired immunodeficiency syndrome (AIDS). There is also a new section on steps people can take to reduce the spread of genital herpes between sexual partners; besides use of condoms, this section discusses exciting new information about how treatment of an infected person with an antiviral drug can reduce the likelihood of spreading the infection to the partner. The section on neonatal herpes has also been updated and new information provided about the use of antiviral drugs during pregnancy to reduce the recurrent infection in the pregnant woman and hence the need for cesarean delivery. The chapter on vaccines has been updated to include new information about a promising herpes vaccine that has proven effective in preventing genital herpes in women. This chapter has also been expanded to include new information regarding topical microbicides, products in development that are intended for vaginal or rectal use to prevent sexually transmitted infections including genital herpes and HIV.

I am indebted to many friends and colleagues who have contributed to our understanding of genital and neonatal herpes from the biomedical perspective, from the psychosocial perspective, and most importantly from the human perspective. Besides those listed in the acknowledgments of the first edition, I would like to recognize Fred Aoki at the University of Manitoba, David Kimberlin at the University of Alabama–Birmingham, Hunter Handsfield at the University of Washington, Gray Davis of Family Health International, Chloe Deleigh of the Technische Universität Gräfenberg, and Pierre Vandepapeliere of GlaxoSmithKline Biologicals–Rixensart. This edition introduces the exciting field of topical microbicide research for the prevention of genital herpes. This field was championed early by Penny Hitchcock of the U.S. National Institute of Allergy and Infectious Diseases. The field continues to advance through the efforts of Caroline Deal of the U.S. National Institute of Allergy and Infectious Diseases, David Phillips of the Population Council, Richard Cone of Johns Hopkins University, Thomas Moench of ReProtect, Inc., Al Profy of Indevus Pharmaceuticals, and Thomas McCarthy of Starpharma. I am grateful to Tony Simmons for his kind contribution of the new electron photomicrograph of the herpes simplex virus that we have used in the second edition. I would also like to thank Ana Ugueto, Ph.D., and Jennifer Yates, M.A., for their assistance in developing the index for the second edition.

Finally, I would like to acknowledge and thank the many patients and their loved ones who have helped me understand herpes.

I would like to thank my friends and colleagues at the Children's Hospital Medical Center and University of

Cincinnati College of Medicine who, over the past fifteen years, have contributed to our research concerning herpes simplex virus infections. They include Martin Myers, David Bernstein, Nigel Bourne, Shirley Reising, Frank Biro, and Susan Rosenthal. I want to acknowledge the important work of some pioneers in the field of clinical herpesvirus research, including Ann Arvin and Charles Prober of Stanford University, Larry Corey, Anna Wald, Rhoda Ashley, and Zane Brown at the University of Washington–Seattle, Steve Straus at the National Institutes of Health in Bethesda, Maryland, Rich Whitley at the University of Alabama at Birmingham, Steve Sacks at the University of British Columbia, Tony Cunningham and Andrian Mindel at the University of Sydney, Steve Kohl at the University of California at San Francisco, Andre Nahmias at Emory University, Moncef Slaoui at SmithKline Beecham Biologicals in Rixensart, Belgium, Rae Lyn Burke at Chiron Vaccines in Emeryville, California, Tsuneo Morishima at Nagoya University, and Phil Krause at the U.S. Food and Drug Administration. I would like to thank Terri Warren of Westover Clinic, Michael Reitano and Charles Ebel of the Herpes Advice Center, and Peggy Clarke of the American Social Health Association for their influential thoughts regarding sensitive psychosocial issues surrounding herpes and the impact of such issues on the lives of people with the disease. I thank Desiree Ellison and Monica Bohlen for their help with the section on herpes and the law. I am grateful to Rick Pyles for his generous donation of the electron photomicrograph of the herpes simplex virus, to Toni Cunningham for help with manuscript preparation, to Margret Richards and Deborah Stewart for help with the glossary, and especially to my colleague Bev Connelly for creating the figures. Thanks go to Miriam Bloom, editor of the Understanding Health and Sickness Series at the University Press of Mississippi, for the opportunity to write this book. Finally, I would like to acknowledge the patience of my family, Elizabeth, Lindsey, and Martin, without whose indulgence I would never have found the time to complete the project.

Introduction

Herpes simplex viruses are remarkably complex microbes capable of causing a wide variety of infections, including genital herpes, a common and chronic sexually transmitted disease. Our understanding of the biology of these viruses has increased enormously over the past three decades, as has our recognition of the pervasiveness of herpes simplex virus infections. Greater awareness of the problems associated with sexually acquired herpes simplex virus infection has led to a better understanding of the disease's psychosocial impact. The availability of new antiviral drugs, used in combination with counselling (when appropriate), now allows for the successful management of most herpes infections. Ongoing research holds promise for the development of vaccines to prevent herpes simplex virus disease and possibly for new therapeutic vaccines designed for the treatment of people already infected.

Sooner or later most Americans become infected with herpes simplex virus type 1, the cause of the common fever blister or cold sore. What is alarming is that more than one out of five American adults have also been infected with herpes simplex virus type 2, the most common cause of genital herpes. Surprisingly, most people with genital herpes are unaware that they have been infected, but even those with no recognizable signs or symptoms of disease can be contagious and spread the infection to a sexual partner. This book was written for people who wish to learn about herpes simplex virus. Readers may include those who have recently experienced their first episode of genital herpes as well as those who suffer from recurrent infections, individuals dating a person with genital herpes, close friends and family members who provide important psychological support to those with the disease, pregnant women with genital herpes or those at risk of getting the infection during their pregnancy, parents of children with neonatal herpes, counsellors and therapists who help people cope with the condition, and people with nongenital herpes infections such as herpes of the eye or lip. This book is also intended for teachers and for health care workers who want to update and round out their information on herpes.

We begin with a look at viruses, the smallest disease-causing microbes. The first chapter, introducing readers to the large family of herpesviruses, explains why there are two different herpes simplex viruses, types 1 and 2, and gives a history of the disease. Chapter 2 discusses the pathogenesis of infection— how the virus actually causes disease, how and where it persists in the body, and how it causes recurrent infections. In the following chapter on epidemiology, we learn how common herpes simplex virus infections are and who is most likely to become infected. Chapter 4, concerned with first episode genital herpes, provides in-depth information about how the infection is acquired, as well as about incubation periods, signs, symptoms, and complications. Chapter 5 contains a detailed discussion of recurrent genital herpes, including topics such as how the disease differs from first episode infection, problems caused by asymptomatic (silent) recurrent infections, prodromes (premonitory symptoms) and false prodromes, and what predicts or triggers recurrences. Next, because herpes simplex virus infections can be especially dangerous under certain circumstances, we discuss infection in immunocompromised persons (those with cancer or AIDS) and pregnant women, and we look at the special problem of herpes in the newborn baby. Besides being painful, herpes infections, especially genital herpes, can cause major emotional problems for the infected person, as well as, occasionally, financial and legal difficulties.

Chapter 7 deals with the psychological impact of the disease and explores ways of coping with it. Information is also given here regarding herpes and health insurance, and we examine the legal ramifications of knowingly infecting another person with genital herpes. Chapter 8 describes the various therapies used in the treatment of herpes infections, from prescription drugs to home remedies, and explains why it is so difficult to prove that a treatment is effective. In the final chapter we review the history and problems associated with making a safe and effective vaccine to protect people against herpes simplex virus infections, and we discuss the idea of therapeutic vaccines, designed for the treatment of people already infected with herpes. For those who want to learn more about herpes or are seeking support groups, the book concludes with several appendices that identify other sources of information.

Understanding Herpes

1. The Herpes Virus, Past and Present

The word "herpes" means different things to different people. To some, herpes is the name given to the troubling blisters or sores that can periodically appear on or around the lips. To others, herpes is a feared sexually transmitted disease that can be caught once but which has a painful aftermath that can be reexperienced many times. The term "herpes" can be appropriately applied to both these common afflictions, but, in addition, medical personnel recognize herpes of the mouth (herpes gingivostomatitis), herpes of the throat (herpes pharyngitis), herpes of the eye (herpes keratitis), herpes of the brain (herpes encephalitis), and herpes of the newborn infant (neonatal herpes). These illnesses are related because they are all caused by the same two closely related viruses, herpes simplex virus type 1 and herpes simplex virus type 2. Viruses, including herpes simplex virus type 1 and type 2, are a major cause of suffering for all living creatures.

What are Viruses?

Viruses are the smallest known microbes or infectious agents. The simplest viruses consist of a core of nucleic acid surrounded by a protein coat known as a *capsid*; this nucleic acid-protein complex is referred to as a *nucleocapsid*. In more complex viruses the nucleocapsid is surrounded by an *envelope*, which is a membrane-like structure containing carbohydrates, lipids and proteins. Viruses contain either *ribonucleic acid* (RNA) or *deoxyribonucleic acid* (DNA), which are large complex chemicals that contain the viruses' genetic code and serve as a blueprint for making more viruses.

Some scientists feel that viruses are not living matter but exist at the border between life and nonlife. This argument is made because, unlike bacteria and more complex organisms, viruses do not carry all the equipment necessary to reproduce themselves. In order to multiply, the virus enters a living cell, removing its protein coat in the process, and then uses its RNA or DNA to redirect the cell's synthesizing machinery to make more copies of the virus. The process of making new viruses can injure or kill the host cell. If enough cells are injured or destroyed, the process results in a recognizable illness such as influenza, viral diarrhea, or genital herpes.

Scientists have identified hundreds of different viruses and there are probably thousands of others still to be discovered. Why do so many viruses exist? Because each is adapted to infect a particular type of cell in a specific living organism. Since there are many different types of cells and thousands of diverse species, thousands of different viruses have evolved. Because they are specialized, some viruses can only infect, for instance, liver cells or muscle cells or brain cells. They are also limited by the type of species they can infect; while some infect humans, others infect reptiles or amphibians or insects or plants or even bacteria. This specificity means that a virus from one animal species, such as cats, usually can't cause infection in a different type of animal, such as dogs. As with most rules, there are exceptions. Some viruses can cause similar diseases in closely related species; for example, varicella virus can cause chicken pox in humans and gorillas but not in their close relative, the chimpanzee. A few viruses can cause comparable illnesses in different species; influenza virus, for instance, can cause respiratory infection in humans, ducks, and pigs (thus, the swine flu).

Physicians and scientists have different approaches to cataloging all of these viruses. Medical doctors generally categorize viruses based upon the type of illness they cause, such as respiratory viruses, hepatitis viruses, and so on. Scientists, on the other hand, classify them based upon physical and chemical properties, like size and shape of the virus particle and type of nucleic acid. Viruses with similar structural and biochemical characteristics are placed in the same family. For example, *rhabdoviruses* (*rhabdos* is the Greek word for "rod shaped") like the rabies virus are rod or bullet shaped and contain RNA, while *poxviruses* (including variola virus, the cause of smallpox) are brick-like or egg shaped and contain DNA. Viruses within a family may infect unrelated species. Within the *hepadnavirus* family are RNA viruses that cause hepatitis in ducks and humans, while other members of the family cause mottling of cauliflower, blueberries, and carnations. Viruses within a family may also cause very different illnesses in the same species. Humans, for instance, can be infected with several different members of the *picornavirus* family, including the polio viruses, which can infect nerve cells and cause paralysis, the *rhinoviruses*, which cause the common cold, and hepatitis A virus, which infects liver cells and causes hepatitis.

The Herpesvirus Family

Herpes simplex viruses type 1 and type 2 are members of the herpesvirus family. (The term "herpesvirus" refers to any member of the family.) For a virus to be a herpesvirus it must have the right shape and contain the right nucleic acid. The capsid of a herpesvirus is in the shape of an icosahedron, a

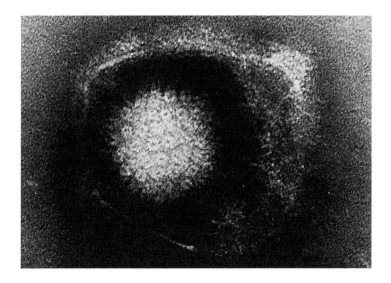

Figure 1.1 Electron micrograph of a herpesvirus (courtesy of Professor Anthony Simmons)

cubic structure having 20 equal triangular surfaces, made up of 162 smaller units called capsomeres. The nucleocapsid contains DNA and is surrounded by an envelope with spike-like structures projecting from the surface (fig. 1.1).

Herpesviruses are complex microbes that produce from 70 to more than 200 specialized proteins that are needed for their reproduction and survival. Because these proteins are important for the virus, but not for the cell, it is theoretically possible that new drugs can be developed that will interfere with the production or function of these proteins. Ideally, such drugs would have no effect on healthy cells but would act on infected cells to block the production and spread of new virus. Scientists are currently studying many of the different herpesvirus proteins in the hope that the information can be used to develop useful new drugs to treat herpesvirus infections.

So far, scientists have identified over 115 different herpes-viruses and have shown that more than 50 different animal species can be infected with some type of herpesvirus. Pigs and turkeys, for example, can be infected with a herpesvirus; species such as rats, snakes, toads, and lizards can spread herpesviruses to their companions. The bottom-feeding catfish and even the majestic bald eagle can be infected. Herpesvirus infections are among the most common contagious diseases in the world.

Of the more than 100 animal herpesviruses, 9 are known to cause disease in humans. One of these viruses, *cercopithecid herpesvirus 1*, also known as B virus, is normally found in monkeys but can cause fatal infection in humans bitten by an infected monkey. Humans are the natural reservoir for the other 8 viruses; that is, these viruses are normally spread from human to human and generally do not cause disease in other animals. In addition to herpes simplex virus types 1 and 2, the other "human" herpesviruses include the closely related *varicella-zoster virus* and the more distant relatives including *cytomegalovirus, Epstein-Barr virus*, and the recently discovered *humanherpes viruses 6, 7, and 8.* Common illnesses caused by these viruses are listed in Table 1.

In the beginning . . .

In the beginning there was only one herpes simplex virus. Millions of years ago, when humans lived in small, isolated clusters, the ancestral herpes simplex virus evolved a strategy for survival. By trial and error (mutation and selection), the virus discovered a way to remain in nerve cells. When herpes simplex virus spread through a village, instead of disappearing after all members of the community were infected, it would

Table 1.1 Human Herpesviruses and Their Common Illnesses

Herpes simplex virus type 1 and type 2

 Genital herpes

 Herpes labialis—fever blisters or cold sores

 Gingivostomatitis—infection of the mouth

 Pharyngitis—infection of the throat

 Keratitis—infection of the eye

 Encephalitis—infection of the brain

 Neonatal herpes—infection of the newborn

Varicella-zoster virus

 Varicella—chicken pox

 Zoster—shingles

Cytomegalovirus

 Infectious mononucleosis-like illness

 Infection of the fetus causing birth defects

Epstein-Barr virus

 Infectious mononucleosis

Human herpesvirus 6

 Roseola

 High fever in young children

Human herpesvirus 7

 Roseola

Human herpesvirus 8

 Kaposi sarcoma

hibernate in the infected persons' nerve cells and periodically reawaken to afflict new susceptible hosts (visitors to the village or the next generation of villagers). In this way, the virus could survive for generations in isolated villages and could spread to other villages via infected travelers. This situation was great for the virus, but the host suffered from illness not only when first infected but also when the virus reawakened.

Based on analogy to the herpesviruses that infect monkeys and the great apes, the ancestral herpes simplex virus is thought to have been capable of causing either oral or genital infection, depending on how the virus was spread. Higher, nonhuman primates exhibit behaviors that allow for the mixing of oral and genital secretions—hence the transfer of virus from the oral cavity to the genital tract and vice versa. Chimpanzees have both direct and indirect oral-genital contact, including oral-genital intercourse, genitalia-to-finger-to-mouth behaviors, autofellatio, and self-stimulation. Adolescent female orangutans orally stimulate the genitalia of adult, male orangutans, while male gorillas perform manual and oral inspection of the genitalia of female gorillas in estrus. Because of these behaviors, the ancestral herpes simplex virus was probably capable of infecting both the oral cavity and the genital tract and was able to hibernate and reawaken from the nerve cells that supplied the mouth or the genitalia.

It is believed that about 8 million years ago, around the time humans and the great apes diverged, the ancestral herpes simplex virus evolved to give rise to two distinct but related viruses: herpes simplex virus type 1 and herpes simplex virus type 2. Two conditions probably facilitated this development. First, as the earliest humans developed a more upright posture, it became difficult for them to put their mouths on their own genitals. This change in behavior would have decreased the mixing of oral and genital secretions, thus somewhat isolating the mouth from the genitals. In nature, such isolation facilitates evolution and probably allowed the two viruses to diverge from their ancestor. The type 1 virus evolved attributes that made it more successful in causing oral infections, while the type 2 virus developed properties that enhanced its survival in and around the genitals. The second circumstance that was important in the evolution of the herpes simplex viruses was probably a change in mating behavior. Most non-human primates (as well as dogs) prefer front to back mating, while some creatures, such as orangutans, prefer front to front mating. It has been suggested that as our earliest human ancestors diverged from the great apes they switched from front to back mating to front to front mating. This change in behavior allowed for more frequent oral-oral and genital-genital contact, which permitted the newly evolving viruses to establish themselves in their particular niche. However, the increase in oral-oral and genital-genital contact brought about by these changes did not eliminate oral-genital contact. Indeed, after millions of years, both herpes simplex virus types 1 and 2 still retain their ability to cause either oral or genital infection. Nevertheless, the two viruses are different in one very important respect. The hibernating type 1 virus is far more likely to cause recurrent oral herpes instead of genital herpes, while the opposite is true for the hibernating type 2 virus, which commonly causes recurrent genital infections but rarely causes recurrent oral infections. This fact suggests that changes occurring through evolution made it easier for the hibernating type 1 virus to awaken from the nerve cells that supply the face than from the nerve cells that supply the genitals, and vice versa for herpes simplex virus type 2.

Early recorded history

The term "herpes," from a Greek word meaning "to creep," was used 2,500 years ago by physicians in the time of Hippocrates to describe spreading skin lesions. This probably included not only herpes simplex virus infections but also other conditions such as ringworm, shingles, and eczema. Richard Morton, in 1694, was the first to use the term to describe what was clearly a herpes simplex virus infection. In 1714 Daniel Turner provided an almost modern description of oral herpes when he wrote, "The herpes is a choleric pustule breaking forth of the skin diversely, and accordingly receiving diverse denomination. If they appear single, as they do often in the face, they arise with a sharp top and inflamed base; and having discharged a drop of the matter they contain, the redness and pain go off and they dry away of themselves."

The French physician Jean Astruc first described genital herpes in men and women in 1736 (before the permissive Napoleonic era). The earliest clear distinction between oral and genital herpes came at the turn of the nineteenth century when Robert Willan and Thomas Bateman, at the Carey Street Dispensary in London, published works describing "herpes labialis" (fever blisters or cold sores) and "herpes praeputialis" (genital herpes). Interestingly, these English physicians did not consider herpes to be a contagious disease. Fever blisters were not shown to contain infectious material until the late nineteenth century, and, in 1921, fluid from genital herpes lesions was demonstrated to be infectious. However, by that time, genital herpes was well recognized as a venereal disease.

In the 1920s, it was discovered that the agents responsible for herpes infections could be grown in rabbits and in chicken embryos. This breakthrough led to the recognition that the virus or viruses responsible for oral or genital herpes could cause other diseases, including infection of the brain (herpes encephalitis), the eye (herpes keratitis), and the newborn (neonatal herpes). While most physicians believed that all herpes infections were caused by one virus, German physician Bernard Lipschutz suggested in 1921 that, while oral and genital herpes were related illnesses, they were nevertheless caused by different viruses. Finally, in 1962 in Germany, Karl Schneweis discovered the fruits of millions of years of evolution when he showed that there were two distinct herpes simplex viruses. Shortly after that, two Americans, Andre Nahmias and Walter Dowdle, showed that most cases of oral and eye herpes were due to the type 1 virus, while the majority of causes of genital and neonatal herpes were caused by the type 2 virus. It is apparent that, despite 10 million years of evolution, humans still mix oral and genital secretions. As a consequence, some cases of oral herpes are due to herpes simplex virus type 2, and, conversely, perhaps 30 percent of the cases of genital herpes in the United States are due to the type 1 virus.

2. How the Virus Causes Disease

Both herpes simplex virus type 1 and type 2 can cause several very different illnesses, including eye infection, fever blisters/cold sores, and genital herpes. At one time, physicians thought that herpes simplex virus type 1 caused infection only above the waist, infecting the lips, eyes and so on, while the type 2 virus infected only below the waist, causing genital herpes. It is now recognized that both types of virus are equally capable of causing infection above or below the waist and that either virus can cause any of the different forms of herpes. The important determinant of first episode disease is not the virus type but rather the anatomic location where the virus enters the body, the so-called portal of entry. For eye infections, the virus must come into contact with the eye; for infections of the lips, mouth and throat, the virus enters through the mouth; and for genital herpes, the infection begins when the virus comes into contact with genital or anal mucous membranes.

The Transmission of Genital Herpes

Most people who get genital herpes become infected when they have sexual intercourse with someone who has the virus, which is transmitted or spread from the infected person's genitals to those of the susceptible individual. One troubling aspect of genital herpes is that a person can be infected and not know it. People with asymptomatic or unrecognized genital herpes can be contagious. *It is, therefore, possible to catch genital herpes from someone who doesn't know that he or she is infected.*

There are ways besides intercourse for the genitals to come into contact with herpes simplex virus. The second most common method of transmission is through oral-genital sex. Most people don't realize that fever blisters or cold sores (herpes labialis) are caused by herpes simplex virus. Millions of virus particles in the tiny sores go wherever the lips take them. Unfortunately, people can also have asymptomatic or unrecognized herpes simplex virus infection of the mouth; they are contagious when shedding virus in their saliva even if they don't have an obvious sore. People who have had an oral herpes infection are estimated to shed virus about 1 day in 20, or around 5 percent of the time. With virus present in saliva or sores, transmission to the genitals can occur from direct contact with lips or tongue or indirectly via fingers that have had contact with the sores or the contaminated saliva. While it is true that herpes simplex virus can live for minutes to hours on inanimate objects, including toilet seats, door knobs, telephones, and surfaces around hot tubs, the likelihood of acquiring a herpes infection from touching such a source is infinitesimally small. Casual contact with a contaminated object is highly unlikely to result in spread of the virus.

The virus life cycle

Coming into contact with the virus is just the first step in a complex series of events that results in genital herpes. What occurs next is an adventure in molecular, cellular, and immune system biology (fig. 2.1).

Projecting from the outer surface of the virus are protein-carbohydrate structures called glycoproteins. At least two of

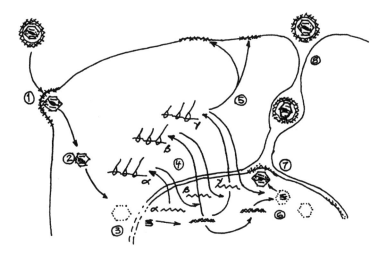

Figure 2.1 Virus replication in a single cell. (1) Attachment and fusion of viral envelope with cell membrane. (2) Microtubular transport of nucleocapsid to nucleus. (3) Release of viral DNA from core and entry into nucleus. (4) Transcription of viral DNA with sequential production of alpha, beta, and gamma gene products. (5) Transport of various viral proteins to cell surface and nucleus. (6) Replication of viral DNA and assembly with viral proteins into new nucleocapsids. (7) Budding of new virion from nuclear membrane. (8) Transport and release of enveloped virus

these structures, glycoprotein B and glycoprotein C, allow the virus to attach initially to proteoglycans. These are complex chemical structures which are present on the surface of living cells. This initial contact is believed to bring other viral glycoproteins into proximity with cellular proteins, allowing glycoprotein D on the surface of the virus to attach to an entry receptor on the cell. Cells were not designed with special receptors to help the virus get inside. Instead, the clever virus developed proteins that can attach to receptors that perform functions important for the cell. The herpes entry receptor probably evolved as a binding site for special growth factors that are produced by the body and play a role in keeping the cells healthy. After stable attachment has occurred, two other viral glycoproteins, H and L, interact with cell surface structures to trigger changes in the cell membrane's cytoskeletal structure. These changes allow the viral envelope to fuse with the cell plasma membrane. In other words, the envelope around the virus flows into the cell membrane in a way that resembles two soap bubbles merging to form one.

When fusion occurs, the nucleocapsid of the virus enters into the compartment of the cell called the cytoplasm. Once inside the cell, the virus attaches to tiny, skeleton-like structures known as microtubules and microfilaments. These structures form an internal transportation network used to move materials within the cell. Using this machinery, the virus moves to the nuclear membrane, where the viral core releases its contents, and the heart of the virus, the DNA, enters the nucleus. The nucleus is designed for storing, reading and copying the cell's DNA. The cell's DNA, or cellular genome, is a genetic blueprint containing all of the information needed for operating or duplicating the cell. When the viral DNA or genome enters the nucleus, it is read by the nuclear machinery and initially makes RNA copies of selected viral genes in a process called transcription. These messenger RNAs leave the nucleus and go to a specialized structure in the cytoplasm known as the *endoplasmic reticulum*. In a process called translation, *ribosomes* in the endoplasmic reticulum read the messenger RNA and assemble the protein encoded by the message. Some of these proteins are subsequently used to help make new copies of the viral DNA; others are structural proteins that are used in constructing new virus cores and envelopes. Through a carefully regulated cascade of transcription and translation, materials for new viruses are produced and assembled into new virus particles, or virions. The new virions are released from the cell and spread to and infect other surrounding cells. Herpes simplex viruses are particularly nasty, and the process of generating new virus particles kills the infected cell. In cells grown in test tubes, the replication of herpes simplex virus from virion attachment to production of progeny virus takes about 18 to 20 hours.

Spreading through nerves

In addition to infecting cells at the portal of entry, herpes simplex viruses can also enter the tiny sensory nerves that are present in the genital skin (fig. 2.2). Sensory nerves are long specialized cells that extend from the skin all the way to the spinal cord. These nerve fibers transmit the sensations of touch, temperature, pain, and position. The nuclei and cell bodies of the sensory nerve cells that supply the genital skin are located in specialized anatomic structures called sacral dorsal root ganglia found near the base of the spine. The mechanism of entry into nerve endings is thought to be similar to that described above for other cells. Upon entry into the nerve ending, the viral envelope is lost and the virion nucleocapsid containing viral DNA moves by means of an axoplasmic transport mechanism along the microtubular cytoskeleton to the nucleus of the neuron located in the dorsal root ganglia. Replication of the herpes simplex virus genome in neurons is thought to occur through a process similar to that which occurs in skin cells, but it requires some specialized viral enzymes, such as thymidine kinase, which are not necessary for virus replication in rapidly growing skin cells. Herpes simplex virus replication in neurons results in the production of nucleocapsids which lack an envelope. The unenveloped

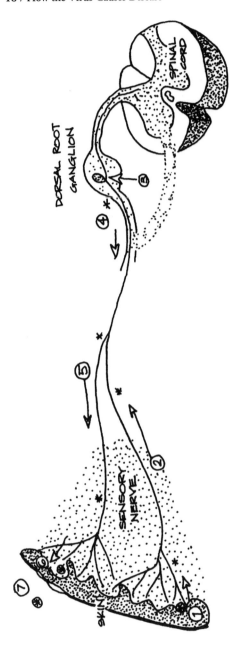

Figure 2.2 The pathogenesis of primary genital herpes. (1) Entry of virus into nerve. (2) Retrograde transport of unenveloped nucleocapsid to cell body within axon of sensory nerve. (3) Replication of virus in neuron within the dorsal root ganglion. (4) Release of progeny nucleocapsids from infected neuron. (5) Anterograde transport of nucleocapsid to skin or mucosal surface. (6) Release of enveloped virus from nerve ending. (7) Replication of virus in skin or mucosal tissue and formation of lesion

nucleocapsids are transported through sensory nerve fibers back to the genital area via a microtubule-associated transport process. There appears to be a separate transport of viral glycoproteins to the nerve ending where the final assembly of the virus takes place. Virus is then released from sensory nerve endings and infects new cells; this action starts the process over again. The replication of virus in mucosal and skin cells and the resulting immune response to the invading virus cause the formation of the small blisters known as herpetic vesicles. Because there is an extensive network of nerve fibers running from the sacral dorsal root ganglia to the skin, virus that enters nerve fibers in the genitals can spread from the ganglia to locations somewhat distant to the portal of entry, including the thigh, buttocks, and anal area. The development of herpetic vesicles around the rectal opening can be due to anal intercourse, but is generally the result of the neural spread of virus from the genital tract to skin around the rectal opening. The intraneuronal movement of virus from the portal of entry to ganglia and back to the skin appears necessary for the production of the herpetic vesicles typically seen with genital herpes.

Unsuspected Cases of Genital Herpes

Not everyone exposed to herpes simplex virus during sexual activity develops genital herpes. Studies measuring antibody to herpes simplex virus type 2 have shown that millions of people are infected with the type 2 virus, but most have never had any signs or symptoms of genital herpes. These people are thought to have experienced subclinical or unrecognized genital herpes simplex virus type 2 infection. Research using animals has shown that the amount or concentration of virus used to infect the animal determines whether the infected animals will develop symptomatic or subclinical genital herpes. There appears to be a minimum amount of virus necessary to initiate the infection of the ganglia, which in turn produces symptomatic disease. At concentrations below the threshold, the virus can infect skin cells at the portal of entry, but the infection does not progress and no recognizable disease develops. It is likely that a similar situation exists for humans and that the amount of virus persons are exposed to also determines whether they develop obvious genital herpes or have an unrecognized or asymptomatic infection.

Prior oral infection with the type 1 virus may reduce the likelihood that a person exposed to the type 2 virus will develop genital herpes disease. People who get fever blisters or cold sores caused by herpes simplex virus type 1 are less likely to develop symptomatic genital herpes if they are exposed to the type 2 virus. In other words, immune responses caused by the type 1 infection can provide some, but not total, protection against getting genital herpes. It is likely that the immune responses present because of the type 1 infection rapidly eliminate some of the type 2 virus, thus reducing the amount of type 2 virus to a level below that necessary to cause symptomatic genital herpes. This protection may work well if the person is only exposed to a small amount of the type 2 virus, but if the amount of exposure is too large, not enough of the type 2 virus can be inactivated and the person will develop symptomatic genital herpes. In general, people cannot know how much virus a sexual partner may be shedding. However, we do know that usually only a small amount of virus is shed from a person who has no symptoms (so-called asymptomatic or unrecognized shedding), while people who are experiencing symptomatic recurrences with herpetic vesicles or ulcers shed larger amounts of virus. This suggests that having sex with someone who is experiencing an obvious herpes outbreak is very risky, although intercourse even during the infected person's periods of asymptomatic shedding can result in a partner's acquiring genital herpes. This is why experts recommend that people with genital herpes use condoms even between outbreaks, as they can never be certain when they are shedding the virus.

How the Body Controls Viral Infections

Humans have evolved complex systems of defense against viral infection. When viruses invade, they trigger the body to produce a variety of different types of immune responses. These responses can be artificially divided into innate immunity and adaptive immunity. The two systems often overlap, interacting and communicating via polypeptides known as cytokines. The innate immune system includes special proteins, which act by attaching to and injuring virus-infected cells, as well as natural killer cells that can recognize and destroy virus-infected tissue, and phagocytic cells, which act as scavengers and attack and destroy invading virus particles. The innate immune system responds promptly, although nonspecifically, to virus infection but does not establish immunological memory.

Adaptive immunity is a more sophisticated system of host defense. The adaptive system uses very small fragments of viral proteins, called antigens, to produce responses that are highly specific for the invading virus. Importantly, adaptive immunity makes a record of the experience, thus establishing immunological memory. This means that the next time the body is invaded by the same virus the responses are rapid and specific and generally can prevent the virus from causing disease. The adaptive immune system consists of specialized white blood cells called lymphocytes. Initial exposure to a virus begins a series of cellular interactions which produces both humoral (i.e., antibody) and cellular responses. After exposure to viral antigens, B lymphocytes make virus-specific antibodies, complex proteins that can bind to and inactivate viruses. The T lymphocytes interact with other specialized cells, such as macrophages, which process and present viral antigens in conjunction with the body's major histocompatibility markers. A subset of the primed T lymphocytes (CD4+ cells) help B lymphocytes make antibody while another group of T lymphocytes (CD8+ or cytotoxic T cells) are programmed to kill cells that are infected by the specific virus.

A complex family of polypeptides known as cytokines are also important in fighting viral infections. These cytokine polypeptides affect and regulate cells of both the innate and adaptive immune systems, allowing them to communicate and coordinate immune responses. In addition, some cytokines, such as the interferons, have the ability to render cells resistant to infection by some viruses, including the herpes simplex viruses.

The first time a person is infected with herpes simplex virus, his or her body responds by making a variety of humoral, cellular, and cytokine responses. These responses limit viral replication by making uninfected cells resistant to infection and by destroying infected cells and virus found outside of cells. When the immune system is working properly, it controls the viral infection, and the infected person recovers. If the immune system is weakened or absent because of a genetic disorder, immunosuppressive drugs used to treat cancer or rheumatic diseases, or AIDS, the infection can be more severe and even life threatening. Considering that most people infected with herpes simplex virus never have a recognizable illness, it is apparent that the immune system is remarkably good at controlling this very common viral disease—remarkably good, but not perfect! One very troubling aspect of herpes simplex virus is its ability to cause recurrent infections in people who seem to have entirely normal immune systems. At this time it is uncertain whether people who suffer from recurrent herpes infections have some very slight defect in their immune systems that allows the virus to escape complete control or whether the virus can produce substances that act locally to impair the immune system and slow its ability to limit virus replication. We do know that stimulation of the body's immune responses against the virus can help control recurrent infections. This fact raises the possibility that vaccines or new drugs can be developed that will help the body's immune system better control this persistent pest.

The Virus that Lasts

With most viral diseases, the immune system can control the infection and rid the body of the virus. Herpes, however, as millions of people know, is not like most viral diseases. As we have seen, the herpes virus has found a way to hide from the immune system by hibernating in nerve cells. When the virus is hibernating, it is in an inactive state that cannot be detected by the immune system. This inactive state is referred to as *latency* or *latent infection*. As discussed earlier, when a person is first infected, the virus enters nerve endings and moves to the nerve cell bodies in the sacral dorsal root ganglia. In most nerve cells, the virus begins replicating. However, for unknown reasons, in some nerve cells the virus does not start the replication process, instead hibernating and establishing a latent infection. Scientists believe that both cellular determinants and viral factors influence whether virus will replicate or enter the latent state. At this time, the cellular and viral processes involved in establishment of the latent infection are unknown.

The latently infected nerve cell contains not the whole virus but only the viral DNA which is stored as long chains or concatamers in the cell's nucleus. During the latent infection the cell doesn't appear to make new copies of the viral DNA but does make messenger RNA copies of one small region of the viral genome. These messenger RNAs are called latency-associated transcripts, or LATs. Laboratory research has shown that the region of the viral genome from which the LATs are made can be removed; the resulting virus is still able to cause disease in animals and establish latent infection in nerve cells. This means that LATs are not required for virus replication, nor are they essential for latency. Other experiments have shown that viruses unable to make LATs rarely cause recurrent genital infections. These findings suggest that the LATs are important for controlling recurrent infections, probably by controlling reactivation of the latent virus.

Latent infection per se does not cause illness. Unfortunately for infected people, latent virus in the dorsal root ganglia can be revived to an active state that produces more virus, which, in turn, causes recurrent herpes. Reactivation of the latent virus can occur for no apparent reason, or it can be triggered by circumstances such as trauma or exposure to ultraviolet radiation. How reactivation occurs is unknown, but the net effect is that the nerve cell begins replicating the virus, producing infectious virus. The process of reactivation may cause tingling or odd sensations in the skin known as a prodrome, an early indication for some people that they will soon experience an outbreak of recurrent herpes. After reactivation, the newly made virus particles are transported from the cell body to nerve endings where they undergo final assembly and are released into the skin. The released virus replicates in skin cells and sometimes causes disease such as herpetic sores, but at other times causes no recognizable symptoms. People with either symptomatic or subclinical recurrent infections shed virus from their skin and therefore are contagious (fig. 2.3).

It is generally believed that, over time, people who suffer recurrent genital herpes will have fewer and fewer outbreaks. Animal experiments have shown that the amount of latent viral DNA in the ganglia also decreases over time. It may be that each reactivation uses up some of the latent virus stored in the ganglia, and that, after a while, there is less latent virus around to reactivate. Under most circumstances, the amount of latent virus in the ganglia is set during the first herpes infection. This means that the pattern of recurrences in people with genital herpes generally does not change if they are reexposed to the virus during sexual activities with someone else who also has herpes. Thus a person who has occasional outbreaks of herpes but engages in sexual intercourse with someone who has frequent recurrences will probably continue to have only occasional outbreaks. Once in a while, however, people can be reinfected with a different strain of the virus and can suddenly find themselves having many more episodes of recurrent genital herpes. For this reason, experts recommend that people with genital herpes use condoms even when having intercourse with someone who also has genital herpes.

Type 1 vs. type 2

Both the type 1 and type 2 herpes simplex viruses are bad insofar as they can both cause severe genital infection. When someone first gets genital herpes, it is impossible to tell from the signs and symptoms whether the infection is due to the type 1 or the type 2 virus. There is, however, a marked difference

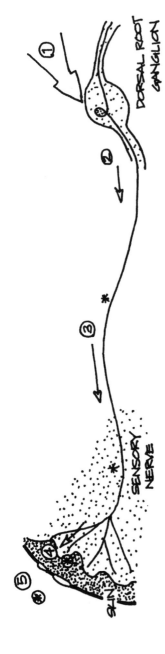

Figure 2.3 The pathogenesis of recurrent genital herpes. (1) Stimulus triggers reactivation of virus in ganglion. (2) Replication and release of nucleocapsids from nucleus of reactivated neuron. (3) Anterograde transport of nucleocapsid to skin or mucosal tissues. (4) Release of enveloped virion from sensory nerve ending. (5) Replication of virus in skin or mucosal tissues and release of infectious virus

in the incidence and frequency of recurrent genital infections caused by these two viruses. The type 1 virus is sometimes viewed as the better of the two, because many people with primary genital type 1 infection never have recurrent infections, and those who do generally have only occasional outbreaks. The type 2 virus is far less kind. Most people with primary genital type 2 herpes do have recurrences, in many cases frequently. Both type 1 and type 2 viruses also produce similar primary infections of the mouth, but recurrent fever blisters are almost always caused by the type 1 virus. Because both viruses are capable of establishing latent infection in sensory nerve cells, it is likely that the two viruses have developed specialized properties that allow them to reactivate more easily in a particular anatomic site—the type 1 virus in the face and the type 2 virus in the genital area. Recent animal studies using genetically engineered viruses showed that the latency associated transcript region of the virus appears to determine the type-specific, site-specific reactivation pattern. Experiments showed that putting the type 1 LAT region in a type 2 virus caused the virus to behave like a type 1 virus. Scientists are now trying to understand how this region controls recurrent disease with the hope that the information can be used to develop new therapies for better control of recurrent herpes infections.

3. Who in the World Gets Herpes

Epidemiology is the scientific discipline that studies the occurrence of disease in populations. One of the main ways epidemiologists estimate how many people have had genital herpes is simply to count all the people with the illness who have been seen in doctors' offices or health clinics. This type of study was done at the Mayo Clinic, where they found that in Minnesota's Olmstead County in 1965, only 1 out of 8,000 people had genital herpes, but, by 1979, the number had increased dramatically to 1 out of every 1,215. This meant that 6 ½ times more people in that county had genital herpes in 1979 than had had it in 1965. This explosive increase in the number of new cases of genital herpes was not limited to Minnesota. The United States government agency that tracks epidemics, the Centers for Disease Control and Prevention, surveyed doctors in private practice throughout the United States and found that there were 10 times more cases of genital herpes in 1984 than in 2003, just 37 years earlier (fig. 3.1).

Some epidemiologists were hopeful that the increase in cases might simply be due to doctors becoming better able to recognize genital herpes. However, over the same time period there was also a large increase in the number of cases of neonatal herpes, an infection usually spread from a mother with genital herpes to her newborn baby. This suggested that the increase in the number of cases of the disease was real—that throughout the 1970s more people than ever were getting genital herpes.

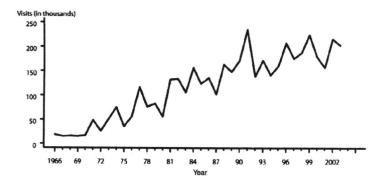

Figure 3.1 Number of people making first-time visits to doctors' offices with complaint of genital herpes, 1966–2003 (Centers for Disease Control and Prevention)

Genital Herpes: an American Epidemic

While counting the number of doctors' patients with genital herpes was a good way to show that more people were becoming infected, epidemiologists realized that this approach would not accurately estimate the total number of people with genital herpes. After all, not everyone with genital herpes could or would seek medical attention; some people had only very mild symptoms that were not troubling, some had symptoms that they did not realize were caused by herpes, and some had no symptoms whatsoever. In order to get a better estimate of how many people were infected with genital herpes, epidemiologists conducted *seroprevalence* studies. When a healthy person is infected with any microbe, his or her body makes *antibodies*, complex proteins that fight the infection. Scientists can develop tests called *assays* to measure specific antibodies in *serum*, the liquid portion of blood remaining after blood clots. Seroprevalence studies determine how many people in any population have antibodies to the microbe of interest. If, for example, 25 percent of a population have antibodies, then it can be concluded that this portion of the population has been infected with the microbe. While this sounds relatively easy, it turned out to be extraordinarily difficult in the case of genital herpes, the reason being that herpes simplex virus type 1 and type 2 are so closely related to each other that the antibody assays could not tell whether a person had antibodies to the type 1 virus, the type 2 virus, or both. This meant that if antibodies to herpes simplex virus were detected, it was uncertain whether the person had type 2 genital herpes or the more common oral infection due to the type 1 virus, or both. The situation was complicated more by the fact that some cases of genital herpes were caused by the type 1 virus, and seroprevalence studies attempting to measure only antibody to the type 2 virus would underestimate the prevalence of genital herpes. Only recently did scientists succeed at making assays that could reliably distinguish between the two herpes simplex viruses. Using one of these assays, the Centers for Disease Control and Prevention conducted a large-scale survey of Americans and found that, in 1978, 16.4 percent of adults had been infected with the type 2 herpes simplex virus. More startling was the finding that by 1990, 21.7 percent of adults had become infected! This discovery was alarming for two reasons: it showed that more than one in five Americans had genital herpes and also that between 1978 and 1990 the proportion of infected people had jumped by 32 percent, a one-third increase in just 12 years. Epidemiologists have found that for every 100 Americans with first-time symptomatic genital herpes, about 85 of the cases will be caused by the type 2 virus, while around 15 cases will be due to herpes simplex virus type 1. Applying these numbers to the seroprevalence data allows us to estimate that *at least 40 million Americans are now infected with genital herpes.*

Why are so many Americans now being infected with genital herpes? Epidemiologists think there may be four reasons for the herpes epidemic. First, people who have had any type 1 virus infection are at reduced risk of getting type 2 genital herpes. Somehow, the body's immune responses to the type 1 virus provide limited protection against becoming infected with the type 2 virus. This means that if you have sexual intercourse with a person who has genital herpes, you will be less likely to get the disease yourself if you have antibody to the type 1 virus. In the past, most people had some kind of type 1 herpes simplex virus infection during childhood. Times have changed, and now many people become adults without ever having had a type 1 virus infection. Without the protective type 1 virus antibody, Americans are more susceptible to getting the type 2 genital infection.

Increased susceptibility alone does not explain why more people are getting genital herpes; the second important aspect of the epidemic is increased exposure. Over the past four decades Americans have begun to have sex at increasingly early ages and with more partners. Both of these behaviors put people at higher risk of getting a sexually transmitted disease, including herpes. It has been suggested that teens postponing first intercourse by 2 years would have a significant impact on the herpes epidemic, as would a reduction in number of sexual partners. We know that men who only have one lifetime partner are at almost no risk of getting genital herpes, while 20 percent of men with 2 to 10 partners will become infected and more than half the men who have 50 or more lifetime partners will get the disease. Women are more susceptible to the infection than men. Given the same number of sexual partners, women are more likely than men to get genital herpes. It is clear that, for men and women alike, having fewer sexual partners is better, or at least safer!

The third factor contributing to the epidemic is the large number of people with asymptomatic or unrecognized genital herpes. As we have seen, these people can be contagious and unknowingly infect their sexual partner or partners. One study of over 5,000 American adults revealed that, among people who had a positive blood test for genital herpes (having anti-body to the type 2 virus in their serum), only 25 percent of whites and 14 percent of African Americans ever had an illness recognized as genital herpes. *This means that fewer than one out of every four people with genital herpes know they are infected.*

The fourth circumstance that may be aiding the spread of the herpes epidemic is the mistaken idea that people are con-tagious only when they have symptoms. It is now well recog-nized by specialists, but not widely known by other doctors or the public, that people who have genital herpes can be conta-gious even when they have no symptoms. This is referred to as asymptomatic virus shedding. In a study of 36 people seen in a clinic for first-time genital herpes, 35 got the infection from genital-to-genital intercourse and 1 from anal-genital sex. At the time of sexual activity, 28 of the people who transmitted the infection did not have any recognizable herpetic sores, nor were any observed by their sexual partners. In this study almost 78 percent of the people spreading genital herpes did not know they were contagious, while in another study nearly 64 percent of the transmitting partners were unaware that they were contagious.

With seroprevalence studies, epidemiologists can determine which groups of people are at greatest risk of getting genital herpes. A study by the Centers for Disease Control and Preven-tion examined the prevalence of genital herpes by sex, race, and marital status. For adult Americans they found that 13 percent of men and 19 percent of women had been infected with herpes simplex virus type 2. Overall, 13 percent of whites and

41 percent of blacks were infected. By marital status, nearly 14 percent of singles had been infected with the type 2 virus, compared to 16 percent of married people and 35 percent of divorced or widowed individuals. A study conducted in Cincinnati found 8 percent of teenage boys and 14 percent of teenage girls had genital type 2 infection. University students appeared to be at low risk, with only around one in fifty testing positive for the type 2 antibody. The lowest risk group, as would be expected, consisted of nuns, all of whom were negative for antibody to herpes simplex virus type 2. The highest risk group, also as predicted, was made up of prostitutes, with almost 4 out of 5 testing positive.

Genital Herpes in Other Countries

Genital herpes occurs in every corner of the world, even in isolated Amazonian Indian tribes. As Dr. Andre Nahmias, a world-renowned epidemiologist, has noted, "The low rate of [herpes simplex virus type 2] antibodies in some isolated Amazonian tribes in Brazil suggests a very recent introduction of the virus by 'civilized' intruders." The type 2 virus obviously travels well. Among the general populations, infection caused by the type 2 virus appears to be most common in the Caribbean, Central America, South America, and Africa, where 20 to 60 percent of the population have been infected. (Seroprevalence studies have been done in Haiti, Costa Rica, Brazil, Zaire, Rwanda, Senegal, and Uganda.) In Europe, fewer people have been infected, in the range of 5 to 30 percent of the population. Limited studies done in Asia show that 6 percent of women in Tokyo, Japan, and 14 percent of women in Taipei, Taiwan, have been infected with the type 2 virus.

Men and Women: Frequency of Occurrence

When epidemiologists conduct seroprevalence studies they consistently find more women than men infected with the type 2 virus. Such a finding suggests that women are more likely than men to get genital herpes. This appears to be true for different groups of women—whites, blacks, teenagers, and so on. Women may be more susceptible to genital infection for two reasons. First, the female genital tract has a greater surface area with more *mucosal cells* (cells that secrete mucus) than does the male *urethra*, the tiny tube inside the penis that carries urine and semen. The mucosal cells are more easily infected than are the *keratinized epithelial cells*, the typical skin cells covering the penis. Second, hormonal changes that occur during the menstrual cycle may interfere with local immune responses, making it easier for the virus to invade a woman's body.

People who have genital herpes want to know what the chances are that they will infect a partner. The spread of genital herpes from a person known to be infected to his or her susceptible partner has been studied in steady heterosexual couples. Doctors have found that about 10 out of 100 susceptible partners become infected each year, meaning that the attack rate or risk of getting or giving genital herpes is about 10 percent per year. The annual attack rate for women averaged 16 percent; that is, 16 out of 100 women whose male partners had genital herpes became infected in one year. For men, fewer than 5 out of 100 became infected in one year, for an annual attack rate of less than 5 percent.

If you are one of the millions of Americans not infected with the type 2 virus and are having sexual intercourse with one of the millions of Americans who has genital herpes, your risk of being infected is reduced if you have antibodies to the other virus, herpes simplex virus type 1. Susceptible persons who have antibodies to the type 1 virus because of a previous nongenital infection like herpes labialis (fever blisters or cold sores) have about a 7 percent per year risk of getting genital herpes; those who have no protective type 1 antibody have about 16 percent per year risk.

If you are susceptible to getting genital herpes, your risk of becoming infected is influenced both by your sex and by your type 1 antibody status. These are two factors that are not easy to change in order to reduce your risk of getting genital herpes. Fortunately, there is something that people can do to reduce their risk of giving or getting genital herpes—*they can use condoms*. In studies of steady couples where one person had genital herpes and his or her partner was susceptible to infection, it was discovered that the spread of genital herpes to the susceptible partner was lower among couples who used condoms regularly.

Not every susceptible person is the steady partner of someone known to have genital herpes. People also want to know what their chances are of getting the disease if they are just average single individuals meeting, dating, and becoming intimate with other single people. Surprisingly, there is only limited information on this important question. A study done by Dr. Andre Nahmais at Emory University in Atlanta found a 2 percent annual attack rate for college students. A study in Sweden found a similar attack rate for women between the ages of 19 and 31. This research suggests that, for the general population, about 2 out of every 100 young, dating adults will get genital herpes each year. A person's overall risk of becoming infected with the type 2 genital herpes virus is influenced by his or her sex, preexisting antibody to the type 1 virus, number of sexual partners, and condom usage.

So, what have we learned from the epidemiologists? First, we see that genital herpes is extremely common; at least one in five American adults are infected. Second, millions of people have genital herpes and don't even know it. Third, people can be contagious at times when they have no signs of the disease. This scenario is pretty frightening, since there is no easy way to know who is infected or when they are contagious.

How to Know if You Have Herpes: Laboratory Tests

There are a variety of reasons people might suspect they have genital herpes. A few days after having intercourse, they might develop for the first time painful small blisters (vesicles) or shallow erosions (ulcers) on their genitals, around their rectal opening, or on their buttocks or thighs. Others might worry about herpes because they periodically experience brief (lasting a few days) episodes of genital itching or changes in the genital or rectal skin such as small red patches or tiny little cracks. Still others might have no symptoms whatsoever but are worried because of their sexual history or that of a sexual partner. In thinking about genital herpes it is important to remember that the clinical findings are highly variable. People who are worried they might have been exposed to herpes or sexually active people who notice periodic changes in the way their genital or rectal areas feel should be checked to see if they have genital herpes—remember more than one in five American adults have genital herpes but most are unaware because their symptoms, the changes in the way their genital or rectal area feels, may be very subtle.

The first step towards determining whether someone has genital herpes is to be evaluated by an experienced healthcare provider. It is best to see the healthcare provider when the person is experiencing the worrisome signs so that the provider can carefully examine the skin and collect samples for laboratory tests. Just a physical examination, even when done by a very experienced clinician, is not always accurate so it is important to *insist* that the clinical diagnosis be confirmed using accurate laboratory tests. The best way to prove someone has genital herpes is to either isolate the virus or detect viral DNA or protein. To do this the healthcare provider needs to see a suspicious change in the skin, preferably a small blister, shallow ulcer, or crack in the skin. The clinician then either rubs or scrapes the suspicious site with a swab or small blade to collect a sample to send to a laboratory for analysis. Pap smears are not useful for detecting herpes because they miss many cases and therefore patients and care providers should not rely on this test when looking for evidence of genital herpes. Depending on the laboratory used by the clinician, the sample collected by rubbing or scraping the suspicious site might be cultured to grow the virus, or it will be tested by PCR (polymerase chain reaction method) to detect viral DNA, or it might be examined under the microscope using immunohistochemical methods to detect viral protein. It may take a few days to a few weeks for the results to be known depending on the test and the laboratory. If the results are positive it is considered proof the person has genital herpes because these tests are generally very accurate. Unfortunately, if the results are negative it does not completely prove the person doesn't have genital herpes because there is always some possibility that the sample sent to the laboratory was not adequate (maybe the clinician did not rub or scrape the suspicious site vigorously enough to get sufficient virus, viral DNA, or viral protein) or was mishandled in transit (maybe it was exposed to 100° temperatures while sitting on a loading dock while being shipped to the laboratory and the high temperature destroyed the virus or DNA or protein). If there are still suspicions that the person might have genital herpes or if the person is seen by their healthcare provider when there are no skin lesions present that can be sampled, then a blood test can be used to look for evidence of infection. These blood tests look for antibodies, infection-fighting proteins which develop within a few weeks of the infection. The main problem with most herpes antibody tests is that they can not distinguish between herpes simplex virus type 1 and herpes simplex virus type 2. This is a problem because most adults have been infected with herpes simplex virus type 1 during their childhood or as teens. Remember, herpes simplex virus type 1 commonly causes infections of the mouth and lips and it is easily spread by sharing things that might be put in the mouth—like a drink glass or a soft drink can—or through kissing (parent-to-child, boyfriend-to-girlfriend, etc.). Some people infected with herpes simplex virus will develop recurrent fever blisters or cold sores on their lips, but millions of Americans have been infected with the type 1 virus and never have any signs of the infection. Remember, most infections with either herpes simplex virus type 1 or type 2 are asymptomatic, that is, the infection is silent and causes no disease.

Fortunately there are two types of accurate blood tests available in the U.S. One is the Western blot test which is provided by the University of Washington's Virology Laboratory. This well-regarded reference test is more expensive and takes longer than most other tests, but it is very helpful if the other tests report that the results are not definitive. More information regarding this laboratory can be found at http://depts.washington.edu/herpes/. The other type of accurate test is referred to as the "gG" test. The test detects antibodies to a herpes simplex virus protein (glycoprotein G) that is different in the type 1 and type 2 virus. Presently there are three gG tests available in the U.S., two of which are made by Focus Technologies of Cypress, California: the HerpeSelect® HSV-1 and HSV-2 ELISA and the HerpeSelect® Immunoblot. The third, the biokit HSV-2 Rapid Test, is available through Biokit, Lexington, Massachusetts. The HerpeSelect® tests are generally run by reference laboratories, although the HerpeSelect® Immunoblot is available at some clinics. The biokit HSV-2 test can be run in about ten minutes and is available at some clinics. These gG tests are all approved by the U.S. Food and Drug Administration.

Be warned, there are many older, inaccurate herpes tests still on the market. Some healthcare providers may not be aware of the recent advances in diagnosing herpes infections and will likely not know which tests are actually performed when they order a herpes simplex virus antibody test. If you or a loved one is going to be tested for genital herpes using a blood test, it is critically important that one of the newer accurate tests be used. One note of caution: about 30 percent of the cases of symptomatic genital herpes disease is caused by the type 1 virus, so testing negative for herpes simplex virus type 2 does not mean that the person doesn't have genital herpes. The only way to prove that someone has genital herpes caused by the type 1 virus is to either detect the virus or viral DNA or protein from a suspicious skin lesion as described at the beginning of this section. The good news is that, unlike genital herpes due to herpes simplex virus type 2, genital infection caused by the type 1 virus only infrequently causes recurrent infections and is spread much less easily through sexual intercourse.

Protecting Against the Spread of Genital Herpes

If you have genital herpes, there are some things you can do to reduce the likelihood that you will transmit the infection to a sexual partner. You can refrain from intercourse during an outbreak and use condoms even when there is no indication that you are experiencing a recurrence. You should be truthful with your partner regarding your infection. Studies show that the spread of herpes is less common when the susceptible partner is aware of the risk. You can also reduce the risk of transmission by using anti-herpes drugs daily. A landmark study found that persons with genital herpes who took valacyclovir daily not only had fewer outbreaks and shed less virus, but were about half as likely to transmit the infection to their partner as those infected persons who didn't use valacyclovir.

4. Genital Herpes: The First Episode

Most people who get genital herpes never have any symptoms; for others, it can be a very painful experience. The first time a person develops recognizable signs and symptoms of genital herpes is referred to as the *first episode*. Subsequent outbreaks are called *recurrences* or *recurrent infections*. Researchers classify first episode genital herpes into three categories: true primary infection, nonprimary infection, and first symptomatic infection. To a person suffering from a first episode, these divisions may seem academic and of little personal relevance. Identifying which category best applies, however, can help determine when the person actually became infected and sometimes makes it possible to predict (or explain after the fact) the severity of the first episode.

What do we mean when we say that knowing which category best fits someone allows the physician to determine when the person actually became infected? People first developing genital herpes assume that the infection was transmitted to them by a partner with whom they have had sexual contact within the past few days or weeks. While generally correct, this is not always the case. In some instances, the person experiencing first episode genital herpes was actually infected months or years earlier, with the virus remaining dormant (latent) in nerve cells and only later reawakening (reactivating) and causing disease. In this situation, the virus causing genital herpes could have been transmitted by a previous partner rather than a recent one. It is important for persons experiencing first episode genital herpes to know that this situation can and does occur, and not to automatically blame their most recent partner for the painful illness they are suffering.

A person with first episode genital herpes is placed into one of the three categories mentioned above based primarily on the results of antibody testing done during the initial illness. A *true primary* first episode occurs only in people who have never had any herpes simplex virus infection before. In these cases, genital herpes can be caused by either herpes simplex virus type 1 or type 2. At the time these individuals become ill with their first episode, they do not have antibodies to either the type 1 or type 2 virus. Because they lack any protective antibodies, they tend to have more severe symptoms and are at increased risk of developing complications. *Nonprimary* first episode genital herpes is generally caused by the type 2 virus and occurs in people who have previously had a nongenital type 1 virus infection such as herpes labialis (fever blisters/cold sores). In these cases, samples taken from the genital sores grow the type 2 virus, but antibody testing shows only type 1 antibodies in the blood. There are no type 2 antibodies initially present, because it takes the body's immune system several weeks to make these specific virus-fighting proteins. Because they have preexisting antibodies to the type 1 virus, people with nonprimary first episode genital herpes may have a less severe illness than does the person experiencing a true primary infection. The third category, *first symptomatic infection*, is almost always due to the type 2 virus. In these cases the initial genital infection was asymptomatic and may have occurred months to years before the person develops what appears to be a newly acquired infection. At the time of the initial infection, the virus moved through nerve fibers from the genital tract to nerve cells in the sacral dorsal root ganglia, where it established a latent infection. For most people who become asymptomatically infected, the virus remains in a latent state forever, and these people never know they have genital herpes. For an unfortunate few, however, the latent virus may reactivate months to years after the initial infection and cause the first outbreak of symptomatic genital herpes. When this occurs, samples taken from the genital sores grow the type 2 virus, and antibody testing also shows the type 2 antibodies present in the blood. Because it takes several weeks for the body's immune system to make antibodies to the invading virus, the presence of the type 2 antibodies at the time the individual first becomes ill indicates that the person was infected with the type 2 herpes simplex virus sometime in the past. The presence of a wide range of preexisting immune responses to the type 2 virus makes the disease caused by a reactivation infection—even a first episode reactivation infection—generally milder than that caused by true primary or nonprimary infections.

Incubation Period

The *incubation period* of a contagious disease is the interval between the time when a person is exposed to a disease-causing microbe and the time when he or she first develops signs and symptoms of the illness. Physicians use the terms "signs" and "symptoms" to describe any abnormality caused by a disease. A *sign* is an objective finding that a doctor can make, for example, a swollen lymph gland. A *symptom* is a subjective finding reported by the patient, as when, for instance, the patient tells the doctor that the swollen lymph gland is tender. For true primary and nonprimary first episode genital herpes, the incubation period ranges from 2 to 20 days, with the average being 6 days. As discussed in chapter 2, it is during the incubation period that the virus enters and multiplies in the cells of the genital tract and also spreads through sensory nerves to the sacral dorsal root ganglia where the latent infection is established. While it may appear that little is happening during the incubation period, this is actually a time of frenzied activity, with the virus spreading and causing injury that will ultimately result in the signs and symptoms of the disease.

Genital Tract Signs and Symptoms

People with first episode genital herpes often experience itching, tingling, burning, and pain in the genital area. In some cases the pain may be so severe that doctors will recommend the use of prescription painkillers. It is not unusual for these symptoms to precede the development of herpetic sores or lesions. *Lesion* is the scientific term for a wound or injury. Herpetic lesions can occur anywhere in the genital area, including on the penis, internal and external aspects of the female genital tract, thighs, buttocks, and around the rectal opening. About 1 out of 10 people with first episode genital herpes also develop herpetic sores in or around the mouth.

On dry skin surfaces like the shaft of the penis, the lesions progress through well-defined stages. The sores begin as *vesicles*, small blister-like lesions usually containing clear or yellow fluid. The skin around the vesicle may be slightly reddened. Because the clear vesicle can be surrounded by reddened skin, some physicians describe the herpetic vesicle as "a dewdrop on a rose petal." After several days, the sores lose the thin skin covering the vesicles and become *ulcers,* shallow erosions in the skin. The skin around the ulcer can also be slightly reddened, with the center of the ulcer having a yellow-gray color. Within a few days the ulcer develops a *crust,* a thin scab covering the sore. The lesions are said to be healed when the crust disappears.

Herpes progresses differently in chronically moist areas such as the *introitus*, the entrance into the vagina. Ulcers are the most commonly seen lesions in these areas. Vesicles do occur but are short lived and rapidly progress to the ulcer stage. Crusts rarely develop; instead, the ulcer slowly fills in with new skin, the process beginning at the edge of the ulcer and moving toward the center. In this fashion the ulcer slowly shrinks in size.

It is important to emphasize that the lesions associated with the first episode of genital herpes are not always like those described in medical textbooks. Herpetic sores can be confused with yeast infection, heat rash, abrasions, jock itch, syphilis, or ingrown hairs. There is also considerable variation in the number of lesions a person will develop. Small lesions may appear to grow together or coalesce to form larger ones. While lesions generally progress from the vesicle stage to complete healing in 7 to 10 days, during first episode genital herpes, people typically have new crops of vesicles developing for the first 2 weeks of the illness. The average duration of lesions—that is, the time from the appearance of the first vesicle until complete healing of the last vesicle to form—is about 16 days for men and 20 days for women. It should be emphasized that there is tremendous person-to-person variability with regard to the duration of lesions. It is estimated that about 1 in 20 people will have lesions for more than 35 days.

First episode genital herpes can also involve the *urethra*, the canal or tube that allows urine to pass from the bladder to the outside. About 4 out of 5 women and 1 out of 4 men with first episode genital herpes develop *urethritis*, inflammation of the urethra usually manifested by a clear discharge or drip and/or by *dysuria*, difficult or painful urination. In some patients with apparently mild skin disease, urination can be extremely painful and may necessitate the use of powerful painkillers.

Most people with primary genital herpes develop swollen lymph nodes in the groin, usually in the second or third week of the illness; this swelling is part of the body's immune response to the infection. While the swelling may be slight, the nodes can be extremely tender. The tenderness and swelling resolve slowly, lasting an average of 9 days in men and 14 days in women.

Generalized Signs and Symptoms

Besides causing painful skin lesions, urethritis, and swollen, tender lymph nodes, the first episode of genital herpes may cause a more generalized illness in about 4 out of 10 men and 7 out of 10 women. For these people, sickness begins as an out-of-sorts feeling, and then develops into a flu-like illness with fever, headache, and muscle pain. This generalized illness lasts 2 to 7 days. *Meningitis*, inflammation of the lining of the brain and spinal cord, develops in 1 out of 10 men and almost 4 out of 10 women with primary genital herpes. The symptoms of meningitis include headache, stiff neck and an unusual photosensitivity, in which normal levels of light cause eye pain. Fortunately, these symptoms last only a few days and patients generally recover completely.

Complications

Candida (yeast) infection is a common complication occurring in more than 1 in 10 women with first episode genital herpes. The symptoms associated with the herpes infection may be improving when suddenly there is an increase in vulvar itching and burning. Some women develop a vaginal discharge or, if they already have a discharge, it may change from thin and watery to thick and cottage cheese-like. Yeast infections complicating genital herpes can be treated with nonprescription products such as Gynelotrimin, Mycelex, or Monostat. An uncommon gynecological complication of genital herpes is *pelvic inflammatory disease*, sometimes called PID. This occurs when the virus spreads above the cervix to involve the uterus and occasionally the fallopian tubes. Women experiencing herpes PID have abdominal pain and a tender uterus. Other sexually transmitted diseases such as gonorrhea and chlamydia are more common causes of PID. If a woman who is experiencing a first episode of genital herpes develops abdominal pain or uterine tenderness she should be checked by a doctor to make certain that she did not get gonorrhea or chlamydia at the same time she became infected with the herpes virus. The drugs used to treat genital herpes also treat herpes PID, but other drugs are required to treat gonorrhea or chlamydia.

Because herpes simplex viruses can invade nerve cells, infection with these viruses can cause nerves to stop working properly. It is common for patients with first episode genital herpes to have changes in sensitivity to touch or pain in or around the genitals. Some people experience increased sensitivity so that even light touch causes tremendous pain. Others have decreased sensitivity or lose sensation entirely in certain areas, which include the lower back, the sacrum or tailbone area, and the perineum, the small triangular region between the thighs that includes the rectal opening and the vulva or the base of the penis. In some people the nerve injury can also cause constipation or problems urinating, and, in some men, it can cause temporary impotence. For the vast majority of people these complications resolve completely within a few weeks.

Other neurologic complications of genital herpes include self-limited meningitis (mentioned above) and *transverse myelitis*, inflammation of the spinal cord that can cause weakness of the legs as well as problems related to bowel and bladder functioning. Most people completely recover from these complications, although there are rare patients who have neurologic problems for years following their first episode of genital herpes.

Some rare complications of first episode genital herpes do occur. In people who have serious problems with their immune system, such as AIDS patients or people taking immunosuppressive drugs for organ transplantation, herpes simplex virus can spread through the bloodstream and cause skin disease that looks like chickenpox. The blood-borne virus can also infect organs and joints, causing pneumonia, liver disease, or arthritis. These complications can also occur in pregnant women, perhaps because their immune system is altered by pregnancy. In people with abnormal immune systems, including pregnant women, these complications can be life threatening. On rare occasions, widespread skin disease with or without pneumonia, liver disease, or arthritis may be seen in people who have apparently normal immune systems.

5. Genital Herpes: Recurrent Episodes

The first episode of genital herpes can be very painful, but eventually the pain subsides and the sores heal. For a lucky few, the only long-term effect of their experience is the slowly fading memory of the pain and discomfort associated with the infection. Most, however, are not so fortunate; soon after the sores of the first episode heal, the majority of people begin to have recurrent genital herpes infections. As discussed in earlier chapters, during the first episode of genital herpes, the virus infects sensory nerve cells in the sacral dorsal root ganglia, setting up a persistent infection referred to as *latency*. Periodically, often for no apparent reason, the latent infection can reawaken or reactivate and cause recurrent infections. With rare exceptions, people do not get recurrent genital herpes because they have been reinfected by their sexual partner; instead, recurrent infections are caused by a virus that is carried in the body, and which can unpredictably reawaken to cause new outbreaks, sometimes over the course of decades! One of the biggest problems with latent herpes simplex virus infections is that they can't be gotten rid of. However, while no medical treatment exists that can destroy the latent infection, there are effective drugs that are useful in treating or preventing the outbreaks.

Recurrent genital herpes can occasionally be as severe as the first episode, with the sores lasting two or more weeks, but most of the time recurrent infections are less painful, with the vesicles and/or ulcers lasting only a few days. For some people the recurrences can be so mild that they may not even be aware they are having an outbreak. Indeed, it is even possible to have an outbreak without having any signs or symptoms whatsoever! These silent recurrences, also referred to as *subclinical shedding, asymptomatic recurrences,* or *unrecognized shedding,* are outbreaks in which the only evidence of the recurrence is the presence of the virus on skin or mucous membranes. Persons having a silent or asymptomatic recurrence are completely unaware that they are having an outbreak. Regardless of whether the episode is asymptomatic or causes painful symptoms, one feature is common to all types of recurrent genital herpes: *a person experiencing recurrent infections is contagious and can transmit the virus to a sexual partner or, very rarely, to a newborn baby.*

Silent or Asymptomatic Recurrences

Doctors have known for almost 20 years that people with genital herpes can shed virus from their genital tract even when they have no symptoms of an outbreak. In the past it was thought that asymptomatic recurrences happened rarely and that with careful training people with recurrent genital herpes could be taught to recognize very subtle symptoms of an outbreak that might otherwise be so mild as to go unnoticed. Indeed, research has proven that people can be taught to notice symptoms of recurrent infection that they previously ignored. But the research also showed that, even with thorough training, people can still have silent recurrences where they shed virus but have no symptoms. It has been long known that people having a recognized outbreak of genital herpes are contagious. What is particularly worrisome is that people experiencing silent recurrences are also contagious. This was dramatically illustrated by a study of 13 *discordant couples,* when a person known to have recurrent genital herpes transmitted the infection to his or her susceptible partner. The study showed that none of the infected people had any signs or symptoms of recurrent genital herpes at the time they spread the virus to their partners. One person had mild symptoms the day before but no symptoms at the time of sexual contact and 3 others developed sores the day after intercourse, but 9 of the people who spread their infection had no signs or symptoms whatsoever.

In the past, doctors told people with genital herpes that they were probably contagious only when they were having a recognizable outbreak. It was thought that if they avoided sexual contact during recurrences they could avoid spreading their infection. It is often distressing for people with genital herpes to learn that they can be contagious even when they have no symptoms. And medical researchers in Seattle, Washington, have shown that silent recurrences occur far more often than was previously realized. In these studies, women with recurrent genital herpes swabbed their genital areas every day for several weeks. In some studies, the swabs were tested by culture for the presence of herpes simplex virus, while in others the scientists used a newly developed and highly sensitive method called *polymerase chain reaction (PCR)* to detect viral DNA. They found that women with primary type 2 virus genital infection had more silent recurrences than did women with a nonprimary type 2 virus infection, while women with primary herpes simplex virus type 1 infection were the least likely to have asymptomatic recurrences. Using the culture method, they found that the average woman with recurrent type 2 virus genital infection had a silent outbreak once every 50 days, but that about 1 in 10 women had a silent recurrence once every 20 days. Most of the time the asymptomatic recurrence lasted only 1 day, but about 1 out of 20 times, the recurrence lasted 4 days or longer, and with no symptoms. Using the ultrasensitive PCR method, which can detect extremely small amounts of the viral DNA, the scientists found that the average woman with recurrent type 2 virus genital infection was asymptomatically shedding virus 1 out of every 4 days! Since we don't know how much virus is required to spread the infection, it is possible that during some asymptomatic recurrences the amount of virus present is so small that the person having the recurrence is actually not contagious. At this time, the best that can be concluded from the recent research is that women (and probably men, too) who have recurrent genital herpes caused by the type 2 virus may have a silent recurrence somewhere between every 4th and every 50th day. This means that asymptomatic recurrences are extremely common. Since these cannot be predicted, the use of a condom, even when the infected person has no symptoms of a recurrence, may be the best strategy for reducing the risk of spreading the infection.

Premonitory Symptoms

About half of all outbreaks of recurrent genital herpes begin with a *prodrome*—that is, premonitory symptoms that occur 1 to 2 days before the development of recurrent lesions. Nine out of 10 people with recurrent genital herpes report that they sometimes have prodromal symptoms. The prodrome may be tingling, itching, or burning in the genital area, or it may be pain, increased sensitivity, or unusual sensations in the groin, scrotum, back, buttocks, thigh, calf, or foot. Occasionally, people describe unusual prodromes such as a metallic taste in the mouth or marked irritability and tiredness. In most cases, the prodromes last less than 24 hours. Scientists believe that the sensations are caused by the reactivation or reawakening of the latent virus present in the sensory ganglia. Movement of the reactivated virus down the nerve and its subsequent replication in skin cells would account for the time between the prodromal symptoms and the development of genital lesions. For some people, the prodrome is a sensitive indicator that they are shortly going to develop genital lesions; however, prodromes are not 100 percent accurate in predicting the onset of recurrent infection. Sometimes people experience so-called *false prodromes*, a situation in which the person notes the telltale prodromal symptoms but fails to develop genital lesions. At this time it is unknown whether a false prodrome represents an aborted reactivation, an asymptomatic recurrence, or the person simply mistaking other sensations for those typically due to a reactivation prodrome.

Signs and Symptoms

While the first episode of genital herpes may be very painful, recurrent infections are more often described as uncomfortable or annoying. It is unusual for people to suffer severely painful recurrences, but it can happen. Except for the local discomfort of the skin lesions and the occasional complaint of a swollen or tender lymph node in the groin area, most people feel relatively well during the recurrent infection, although a small number of people report that they get headaches or feel generally tired. Classically, recurrent infections begin with the development of a discrete reddened area, referred to as *erythema*, which progresses over several hours to form one or more vesicles. A typical recurrence may consist of a single vesicle or of multiple (usually fewer than 10) vesicles grouped together in a small cluster. For some people, new crops of vesicles may erupt at the same site over several hours or over a few days. Less commonly, vesicles may form at one site, and then later a crop of new vesicles may develop at a different site as the first cluster of lesions begins to heal. As with primary infection, the vesicles usually progress to become shallow ulcers that heal by growing new skin from the outside edge in. The average time from when the vesicle appears to complete healing is about 10 days, although there is tremendous individual variation, with the range being 4 to 29 days. It is important to realize that not all recurrences are "typical." Some people only develop (or recognize) ulcers. In women the ulcers can be very small and shallow and found between skin folds, especially in chronically moist areas. At the other end of the spectrum are the large and sometimes painful ulcers that can be mistaken for the sores called *chancres,* which can be caused by syphilis. As stated earlier, the herpes lesions can sometimes be confused with ingrown hairs, heat rash, yeast vaginitis, minor trauma, contact dermatitis, or a variety of other skin conditions. People who have had genital herpes should be aware that any unusual skin lesion or rash in the groin area might be a herpes outbreak. Anyone uncertain about the skin condition should consult a medical specialist.

Unusual Manifestations and Predictors of Frequency

In rare cases, people with recurrent genital herpes have particularly severe or unusual manifestations, which are disturbing for the person and often perplexing for the health care provider. Examples include a sudden increase in the number of recurrences after the virus has been dormant for years, significant problems with urination, severe genital itching, and excruciating pain with the outbreak or chronic postherpetic neuralgia, which is pain that is persistent and sometimes worse in particular positions, such as sitting. People who have severe or unusual recurrences should be evaluated by a health care specialist to be certain there is not some other explanation for their signs and symptoms. Those who are not helped by an antiviral drug like acyclovir may consider consulting a specialist in pain relief. At this time there is no scientific or medical explanation as to why some people experience such unusual or severe recurrences.

Numerous factors probably influence whether a person will have only an occasional recurrent genital infection or will suffer frequent recurrences. Many of these likely determinants, such as how much virus they were exposed to when they became infected, or whether the virus they are infected with is unusually virulent, cannot be studied in people. Consequently, our understanding of what influences the pattern of recurrent infections is very limited. It is known that virus type significantly affects the risk of having recurrent genital herpes. People with genital infection caused by herpes simplex virus type 1 have far fewer recurrences than people infected with herpes simplex virus type 2 (see chapter 2 regarding our limited understanding of this interesting biological phenomenon).

Two factors recognized to influence recurrence patterns are sex and severity of the initial infection. Overall, men have more recognized recurrences than women (the reason for this is unknown). People who have extremely severe initial infections, those lasting more than 35 days, also tend to have more recurrences.

It is surprising that certain factors do not influence how frequently a person will have episodes of recurrent genital herpes. Prior herpes simplex virus type 1 nongenital infection, such as a fever blister or cold sore on the lip, reduces the likelihood that a person will get type 2 genital herpes; however, previous type 1 infection does not influence how many episodes of recurrent genital herpes the person will experience. In other words, people who get fever blisters will have about the same number of recurrent genital infections as people who don't get fever blisters. Also, treatment of the initial episode of genital herpes with acyclovir, an effective antiviral drug, does not decrease the number of recurrent infections the individual will later experience. It might be that acyclovir does not interfere with the establishment of the latent infection, or that by the time the patient starts drug treatment the latent infection is already established.

Factors Triggering Recurrent Genital Infections

Little scientific information exists regarding what can cause the latent virus to reactivate and cause recurrent infections. People who experience recurrent genital herpes report a variety of trigger factors that seem to bring on an outbreak; these include emotional stress, physical exhaustion, lack of sleep, poor nutrition, menstruation, physical trauma, illness, and sun exposure. Irritation or friction at the site of the infection caused by sex or other physical activities like bicycle riding or exercising have also been reported to provoke recurrences. Few studies have carefully examined whether any reported trigger factor actually causes recurrent infections, although survey data indicate that most people believe that stressful events contribute to their herpes outbreaks. People benefit from regular exercise, good nutrition, adequate rest, and stress reduction, regardless of whether these are important in the control of recurrent herpes. At the very least, a healthy life style will help individuals better cope with an outbreak, and for some it may reduce the likelihood that they will experience a recurrent infection.

Genital Herpes and HIV Susceptibility

There is growing evidence that persons with genital herpes are more susceptible to acquiring HIV infection through sexual intercourse. Research suggests they may be three times more susceptible than persons who do not have genital herpes. Two possible explanations have been proposed: (1) that tiny, possibly microscopic breaks in the skin caused by recurrent genital herpes allows HIV easier entrance to the body; or, (2) that the body responds to recurrent outbreaks by sending white blood cells to the genital tract to fight the herpes infection and that HIV infects some of these white blood cells and uses them to gain entry to the body. Studies are underway to determine whether the daily use of antiherpes drugs like acyclovir, famciclovir, or valacyclovir can reduce the risk of contracting HIV infection. At this time, the best approaches for reducing the risk of acquiring HIV are abstinence, monogamy, and condom use.

6. Herpes and Special Situations

Most herpes simplex virus infections are self-limited, meaning that, even without treatment, the herpetic sores eventually heal and the patient recovers. In some situations, however, the infection may be particularly severe or even life threatening.

The Immunocompromised Patient

The body's immune system, described in chapter 2, is important in controlling herpes simplex virus infections. The cellular arm of the immune system, which includes the white blood cells called lymphocytes, is particularly important. Patients with diminished, impaired, or absent cell-mediated immunity are described as being *immunocompromised*. These individuals have a difficult time controlling the virus and are more likely to have severe herpes infections.

Rarely, people are born lacking part of their immune system, an example being those with severe combined immune deficiency (SCID). Individuals with such congenital disorders are often identified in childhood. Impairment of the immune system more often occurs as a consequence of infection, drug treatment, or exposure to ionizing radiation. Infection due to human immunodeficiency virus (HIV) causes a slow destruction of key components of the cellular immune system. Progression of the infection eventually leads to the acquired immune deficiency syndrome, AIDS. Similarly, the ionizing radiation or potent drugs used in the treatment of cancer can damage or destroy the immune system. Patients who receive organ transplants are treated with drugs specifically designed to suppress their immune system so as to reduce the likelihood that they will reject the transplanted organ. Potent immunosuppressive drugs are also used in the treatment of severe collagen vascular disorders like lupus. Finally, people taking very large doses of steroids for any condition may have some impairment of their immune system. Any of these conditions may predispose the patient to have more severe herpes infections, and the more impaired the immune system is, the greater the likelihood is that the infection will be serious or even life threatening.

The immunocompromised patient with either oral or genital herpes may have recurrences that spread to involve large areas of skin. These recurrences generally persist for a much longer time and may cause extensive tissue destruction. Virus present in the recurrent lesions may spread to involve adjacent structures. Patients with herpes labialis (fever blisters) can develop infection of the esophagus, trachea, and/or lungs. For those with genital herpes the infection may extend to involve the uterus, epididymis, or rectum. In rare cases the virus may enter the bloodstream and cause serious coagulation problems. The virus in blood may spread to the liver or adrenal glands, causing hepatitis or adrenal failure. Herpes simplex virus infection of the esophagus, lungs, blood, liver, and/or adrenals is extremely serious and can be fatal.

Another problem experienced by the immunocompromised patient is subclinical viral shedding. While this is also a problem for people with a normal immune system, recent studies suggest that the immunocompromised patient has an increased rate of asymptomatic shedding and thus may be more contagious than people who have an intact immune system.

Because of the potentially life-threatening nature of herpes infections in the immunocompromised patient, these individuals should be cared for by a medical specialist familiar with the problems herpes can cause in this special group.

The Pregnant Woman

Genital herpes can pose special problems for the pregnant woman. In most cases, infections in pregnant women do not differ from those seen in other women; however, primary infections during gestation can be unusually severe and, on occasion, life threatening. This is because pregnancy can depress the immune system, which allows the virus to spread, causing more extensive disease. Perhaps the most dramatic example of severe infection in pregnancy is the rare case of blood-borne dissemination in which the woman develops vesicular lesions over most of her body in an illness that mimics severe chickenpox. Because the initial genital infection is associated with increased complications during pregnancy, any pregnant woman thought to be experiencing the first episode of genital herpes should seek medical care without delay. Most episodes of genital herpes in pregnant women are recurrent infections. These may be clinically apparent or asymptomatic, and they tend to occur more frequently, although the recognized recurrences are typically no more severe than those seen in nonpregnant women.

Genital herpes simplex virus infection can also affect the length or term of the pregnancy. Primary genital herpes in the first trimester has been associated with spontaneous abortions but does not appear to cause birth defects and, therefore, is not a reason to consider termination of the pregnancy. Primary infection in the late second or third trimester has been associated with premature onset of labor and, on occasion, birth defects. Recurrent genital herpes does not appear to cause either spontaneous abortions, premature onset of labor, or birth defects.

Another major problem associated with genital herpes in pregnancy is the potential for the mother's virus to spread to the fetus during gestation (*intrauterine infection*) or to the newborn infant during delivery (*intrapartum infection*). It should be emphasized that spread of herpes from the mother to the baby occurs rarely. As discussed in chapter 3, among the millions of pregnant women who have genital herpes, only a few thousand babies become infected yearly. Intrauterine infection is very uncommon and almost always due to primary genital herpes. It occurs when the virus spreads to the fetus either by ascending from the mother's lower genital tract to her uterus and the placenta or by entering the mother's bloodstream and spreading to the placenta. Intrauterine infection in early pregnancy can cause fetal death, while infection later in gestation may produce birth defects including scarring of the skin, eye abnormalities, and problems with brain development.

Intrapartum infection is 10 to 20 times more common than intrauterine infection. It occurs at or near delivery when the baby is exposed to virus present in the mother's herpetic lesions or infected secretions. The likelihood of intrapartum transmission depends largely on whether the mother is experiencing primary or recurrent genital herpes. The highest risk of transmission (up to 50 percent) occurs when an infant is delivered vaginally to a woman experiencing symptomatic, primary genital infection. The lowest risk (less than 4 percent) exists for the infant exposed to an asymptomatic, recurrent infection. The reason for the big difference in risk probably has to do with how much virus the baby is exposed to and whether the baby has antibody against the virus. Mothers with recurrent genital herpes have antibody in their blood, and these virus-fighting proteins are transferred to the fetus during the pregnancy. Women who have a primary infection need weeks to months in order to make the antibody; hence, their infants are usually born without these virus-fighting proteins. It is thought that exposure to higher viral loads, which are present during a primary infection, increases the risk of transmission, whereas the presence of the passively acquired antibody decreases the risk.

Currently there are two approaches to reducing the risk of intrapartum transmission: delivery of the infant by cesarean section and daily use of anti-herpes drugs by the mother in the last four weeks of the pregnancy. *Cesarean section* is a surgical procedure that involves making an incision in the woman's abdomen and uterus and delivering the baby through the incision. If the mother is recognized to be having an episode of genital herpes (primary or recurrent), the infant will usually be delivered abdominally, regardless of how long her membranes have been ruptured. This is done to avoid intrapartum exposure that can occur if the baby is delivered vaginally through an infected birth canal. However, this approach has many drawbacks. Cesarean section is a surgical procedure that is expensive, causes pain or discomfort, requires some time for recovery, and can be associated with both short-term and long-term complications. Also, delivering a baby by cesarean section does not guarantee that it was not exposed to the virus before the procedure. Because herpes in pregnancy is common but infection of the baby is rare, many women have to undergo cesarean section in order to prevent just one case of neonatal infection. That is why it costs society about $2.5 million to prevent each death of a newborn from herpes simplex virus infection. There is, however, an even greater cost in terms of human life, with about 4 mothers dying of complications resulting from cesarean delivery for every 7 babies saved from herpes-related deaths.

Because of the problems associated with the cesarean section, the use of oral anti-herpes drugs like acyclovir and valacyclovir have been used in the last few weeks of pregnancy in women with a history of recurrent genital herpes to reduce the likelihood the woman will have a recurrent infection at the time of delivery. This approach has reduced the need for cesarean sections by reducing clinically observable recurrent infections, but the question remains as to whether the treatment actually prevents transmission, since intrapartum spread can occur even with subclinical or asymptomatic recurrences. And it should be emphasized that a drug taken by a pregnant woman also reaches the developing fetus. A registry of patients who received acyclovir during their pregnancies found no evidence that treatment caused adverse fetal effects.

Preventing Genital Herpes During Pregnancy

If a pregnant woman's sexual partner is thought to have herpes, he should be tested using one of the new accurate blood tests (see chapter 8). If the partner has genital herpes, there is a chance of spreading the infection to the pregnant woman even when there are no signs or symptoms of active disease. This occurs through asymptomatic shedding (see chapter 2). There are some steps that can be taken to reduce the risk of the pregnant woman becoming infected. The best approach is abstinence—no sexual intercourse or genital-to-genital contact during the pregnancy. If there is to be intercourse, then the use of condoms may reduce but not eliminate the risk of spreading. Also, the daily use of 1 gram of valacyclovir by the infected male partner has been shown to reduce spreading to a non-pregnant susceptible partner. While this approach has not been tested in preventing spreading during pregnancy, it should theoretically work—remember, however, that this approach reduces the likelihood of spreading but may not entirely prevent it.

The Newborn Infant

The term *neonate* refers to an infant in the first month of life. Between 1,000 and 4,000 cases of neonatal herpes simplex virus infection occur each year in the United States. Infection of the neonate can be caused by either the type 1 or type 2 virus. While neonatal herpes can result from the baby being infected in the first few weeks after delivery by someone with a nongenital infection such as herpes labialis (fever blisters), neonatal infection is typically a complication of maternal genital herpes (discussed above). About half the cases of neonatal herpes result from first episode genital infections occurring in the mother around the time of delivery. Amazingly, the initial genital infection is asymptomatic in two-thirds of these women. Approximately 30 percent of the cases of neonatal herpes are due to maternal recurrent genital herpes infection. As with first episode genital infections, two-thirds of these are asymptomatic.

Neonatal herpes is a potentially life-threatening illness. Some newborns have signs and symptoms of infection at birth, but infants typically become ill one to three weeks after delivery. Based upon the results of physical examinations and laboratory tests, neonatal herpes can be divided into three categories: (1) disseminated infection involving multiple organs including brain, lung, liver, adrenal glands, skin, or eyes, (2) central nervous system infection (*encephalitis*) with or without skin infection, and (3) localized skin infection. Recent studies using new and highly sensitive polymerase chain reaction (PCR) tests have shown that some infants who appear to have only local- ized infection actually have disseminated and/or central nervous system infection. It is critically important that any infant thought to have neonatal infection be evaluated by a health care provider without delay. The only effective treatment for neona- tal herpes has to be given intravenously, and early treatment appears to result in a better outcome, especially for localized infection. If the infection begins with localized disease but the baby does not receive treatment, the infection generally prog- resses to disseminated infection and/or encephalitis.

The most severe form of neonatal herpes is the dissemi- nated infection, which occurs in about 20 percent of the infected infants. The baby with disseminated infection may have an abnormal body temperature; some will have a fever, while others may have a temperature that is below normal. Signs and symptoms may also include irritability, lethargy, labored breathing, respiratory distress, cyanosis (bluish or purplish skin caused by lack of oxygen), feeding problems, and seizures (convulsions). Even with treatment, about half the infants with disseminated neonatal herpes will die, and about half the survivors have long-term complications such as mental retardation, blindness, seizures, and behavioral problems.

About one-third of infants with neonatal herpes will have an infection of the central nervous system. These babies may be unusually irritable, may have seizures, or may be lethargic or even unarousable (comatose). Approximately 15 percent of babies with encephalitis die, and more than half of the sur- vivors have some sort of long-term neurologic complication such as slow development, recurrent seizures, blindness, deaf- ness, mental retardation.

The most common form of neonatal herpes is infection that is limited to the skin, eye, or mouth. Localized disease is seen in about half of the infected infants, and with appropriate treatment almost all these babies survive. The most common finding in localized infection is a skin rash composed of vesicular lesions, typically 1–2 mm (.04 to .08 inches) in diameter and usually surrounded by a red (erythematous) halo. Just as with other herpes simplex virus infections, the virus establishes a latent infection in sensory ganglia which can reactivate to cause recurrent infections (see chapter 2). About half of the babies with localized infection will have at least one episode of recurrent herpes within the first six months of life. Approximately 5–10 percent of infants will have more than three cutaneous recurrences in this time period, and these babies are much more likely to have some type of neurologic problem.

There are many problems related to identifying and treating the infant with neonatal herpes. For one thing, fewer than 1 in 3 babies with neonatal infection are born to women known to have genital herpes. That means that even if every woman with recognized genital herpes at the end of pregnancy was delivered by cesarean section, we would reduce the number of cases of neonatal infection by less than 33 percent, and the cost in terms of maternal injury and death would be staggering! Another problem is that the signs and symptoms of neonatal herpes are nonspecific (that is, many illnesses can cause the same clinical findings), and the resulting delays in starting effective therapy may lead to a poorer outcome. Even if therapy is started promptly, not all babies survive, and many who do have permanent injuries. Hence, there is need for better, more effective treatment. In the long term, the best strategy for preventing neonatal herpes will be to prevent genital herpes in the pregnant woman. It is hoped that the development of a vaccine that could prevent genital herpes would also result in a significant reduction in the number of cases of neonatal herpes.

7. Sex, Lies, and Herpes

The psychological and social aspects of genital herpes simplex virus infection are at least as complex and confusing as the virus's molecular biology. This chapter touches on three important areas: the psychological impact of the illness, herpes and the law, and herpes and health insurance. It is important for those concerned about any of these areas to seek additional information from a variety of sources. The well-informed person is best equipped to deal effectively with psychological and social problems that can be associated with genital herpes.

The Psychological Impact of Genital Herpes

The first episode of genital herpes may produce a bewildering array of emotional reactions, including shock, confusion, fear, anger, and feelings of betrayal in those who realize that they have acquired a sexually transmitted infection. After a person recovers from the first episode, the emotional impact of genital herpes mostly results from his or her concerns about the unpredictable recurrent nature of the disease and about possible transmission of the infection to another sexual partner, or, in the case of the pregnant woman, to her baby.

People with genital herpes may view themselves differently from how they did before they acquired the infection. Some people suffer loss of feelings of self-worth, and some report they feel "unclean" or "undesirable." These changes in self-image may lead to depression, with myriad possible manifestations. Some individuals become withdrawn, even from their closest friends. Others, feeling betrayed, end long-term relationships, a distressing outcome since transmission of the virus is not always a clear indication of infidelity. As discussed elsewhere in this book, it is well documented that people can have unrecognized genital herpes and carry the virus for years before transmitting it to a sexual partner. Fear of rejection by future romantic interests causes some to remain in unhappy or even abusive relationships and prevents others from seeking and establishing intimate connections. A few are so distressed by the infection that they experience self-destructive thoughts. The psychological impact of genital herpes is usually greatest in the 12 months following the first episode. The daily use of acyclovir, valacyclovir, or famciclovir to prevent recurrent outbreaks, especially during the first year after acquiring genital herpes, has been shown to improve the patient's quality of life in terms of the impact of the diagnosis. Most people eventually learn to cope with their illness, although a small number with genital herpes report emotional difficulties even years after first acquiring the infection.

Aside from the first episode, genital herpes is rarely a serious illness. While there are people who suffer severe, atypical recurrent infections, and, while transmission to the newborn can have devastating consequences, for the most part genital herpes is a nuisance disease. Why then does it have such psychological impact? The answer resides in our society's conflicting attitudes about sexuality and sexual activity. Americans are constantly bombarded by sexual innuendo that has a profound effect on the defining of our self-image. Sexual desirability and prowess are given very positive connotations, while at the same time society portrays sexual activity as dirty. Most people learn to balance these contradictions, especially in the context of romantic love. Unfortunately, a sexually transmitted disease like genital herpes can disturb this tenuous balance and in so doing negatively affect an individual's self-image; it is this change, more than the physical aspects of the infection, that causes the emotional distress. With time and appropriate support the person with genital herpes can usually reestablish a healthy self-concept.

The emotional distress caused by genital herpes is highly individual, but there is some general advice that should be considered by those learning to cope with the psychological impact of the illness. First, it is important for the person with herpes to have accurate, up-to-date information regarding the infection, including how it is spread and how it can be treated. There is a surprising amount of inaccurate information regarding genital herpes, and even some physicians are not well informed on the subject. A knowledgeable health care provider can be an important resource. An excellent source of regularly updated information is *the helper*, a newsletter published quarterly by the American Social Health Association. A short list of recently published books on genital herpes is also included in appendix B; beware of older books that have not been recently updated, because they may contain inaccurate information. The Internet can be a useful source, although the accuracy of the information presented at different Web sites varies greatly (see appendix C).

Another important element in coping with genital herpes is emotional support. Talking to a trusted confidant about the physical and psychological impact of the illness can reduce the feelings of isolation and rejection. Reassurances from a close friend, family member, health care provider, cleric, or teacher can help place the illness in a proper perspective. Local support groups can be useful in helping the person with recently diagnosed genital herpes to find more experienced people who have developed successful strategies for dealing with their illness. Support groups can also be important in identifying local health care providers who are both knowledgeable and sympathetic regarding genital herpes. Some people report dissatisfaction with their healthcare providers especially in connection with their first visit for this particular problem. The diagnosis can come as a great shock, and sometimes physicians may seem callous. It is important to recognize that, while genital herpes is an extremely common disease, most healthcare providers have limited experience in managing patients with the illness. The problem is further compounded by the small amount of time allocated for the average office visit, typically less than ten minutes. This is hardly sufficient time to evaluate the patient, establish the diagnosis, prescribe treatment, and discuss the immediate and long-term consequences of the illness. Many people are overwhelmed by the diagnosis, and at the initial visit would be in no condition for a lengthy discussion about genital herpes even if more time were available. As with any chronic condition, the person should see the healthcare provider again to discuss the illness and ask whatever questions have arisen. For some it is a good idea to bring a written list of questions to ensure that nothing is forgotten. Persons who, after repeat visits to a clinician, remain unsatisfied with the help they are receiving should find a different health care provider, since professionals can be a very important source of information and support.

A healthy life style also helps in dealing with the emotional aspects of herpes. People who are rested, well nourished, and physically fit cope better with all forms of stress. Everyone, not just those with herpes, benefits from a balanced diet, limited consumption of alcohol and caffeine, and avoidance of tobacco. Regular exercise not only contributes to physical fitness but can significantly improve self-image.

For many people, knowledge, emotional support, and a healthy life style provide the tools necessary to cope with the psychological impact of genital herpes. Help from a mental health professional should be considered when genital herpes has become a major focus of the person's life, when someone feels that the emotional aspects of the illness are overwhelming, or when the individual shows signs of persistent depression. These professionals can offer a variety of treatment options, such as counseling, biofeedback, hypnosis, and psychotropic drug therapy, which can be helpful in dealing with issues of self-esteem, pain management, stress reduction, and interpersonal relationships, including how to discuss genital herpes with a new partner. Although they have not been studied scientifically, stress reduction techniques might also be helpful for persons who perceive that their episodes of recurrent genital herpes are triggered by stress.

One of the biggest problems experienced by many with genital herpes is how to discuss the subject with a new romantic interest. Some fear rejection so much that they either avoid developing intimate relationships or they do not tell their new partners about their history of genital herpes. Both of these situations should be avoided. While some individuals do experience rejection after telling a new companion about their genital herpes, many find that being forthright about their past is the first step in establishing an honest, intimate relationship. Furthermore, there is evidence that telling a partner about having genital herpes actually reduces the likelihood the partner will become infected. Since more than 1 in 5 Americans have genital herpes but most don't know it, a new partner should probably be tested using the newer accurate blood tests to determine whether he or she is already infected. Keeping one's history of this disease secret from a new sexual partner is fraught with problems. It can be even more difficult to share the information later. There are legal implications if the new partner should contract genital herpes, and the secrecy can actually create more anxiety and stress than the truth. How and when such personal information is shared should be carefully planned. Generally the subject should not be brought up until the individual with herpes feels quite comfortable and compatible with his or her new companion. It is important that the person feel self-confident and recognize that herpes is only a small part of life. The information should not be conveyed with a heavy negative emphasis but with the expectation that the new companion will be understanding and supportive. If rejection does occur, it is likely that the relationship would not have evolved into a loving, mutually beneficial, long-term arrangement even if herpes had not been an issue. Because the question of how to discuss the disease with a potential new partner can be difficult, individuals with genital herpes are encouraged to discuss strategies with doctors or nurses at sexual health clinics, mental health specialists who deal with interpersonal relationships, or the professionals at the Herpes Resource Center or Herpes Advice Center.

The Law

Some states, including New York, California, and Ohio, have specific laws (statutes) concerning the spread of contagious diseases. In such states a person may be criminally liable for transmitting genital herpes. Recent court decisions have also established civil liability in cases where people with genital herpes transmit the infection to a sexual partner. Since few states have specific laws dealing with genital herpes, the principles of common law have provided the basis for these successful lawsuits. Common law, based on traditional legal and ethical principles, is continuously evolving as the courts interpret the law in the context of changing social policy. In general, the common law of tort liability is intended to punish wrong-doers, deter wrongful conduct, compensate the victim, and implement society's shared concepts of fairness. It has been argued by some legal scholars that imposing tort liability is an effective means to help control the spread of genital herpes, but since most people with the disease are unaware that they are infected (let alone contagious), it is unlikely that anything the legal system can do will significantly affect the spread of the current epidemic.

The courts have most commonly recognized three causes of action in cases involving transmission of sexually acquired infections: negligence, battery, and misrepresentation. Negligence cases are based on the concept of duty, with the expectation that people with genital herpes are obligated either to avoid sexual contact with uninfected persons or at least to inform their sexual partners about the disease. Once a court recognizes the existence of a duty to protect against transmission of genital herpes, negligence occurs if the defendant fails to refrain from sexual conduct or to disclose the fact that he or she has genital herpes and if the defendant's conduct (in this case sexual intercourse) results in injury to the plaintiff, i.e., that person's acquisition of genital herpes with the resultant physical pain and suffering, emotional trauma, and prospects for long-term complications. Because people with genital herpes may be contagious at times when no symptoms are present, they are obligated to make full disclosure at all times and not just when they realize that they are experiencing episodes of recurrent disease. Disclosure should occur before the onset of sexual activity, with the extent of warning being determined by the sophistication of the partner. In general, for sexually experienced people, the statement that one has genital herpes should fulfill the disclosure requirement. In the case where a person with genital herpes informs his or her sexual partner about the illness and the partner understands the risk and voluntarily proceeds with sexual activity, the partner assumes the risk, and liability will probably not ensue in the event of transmission of the infection. The burden of protecting the partner rests with the infected individual, and, in most cases, the at-risk partner is not obligated to inquire regarding the other person's sexual health.

Battery is intentional and harmful contact with another. In this situation, the sexual activity between partners constitutes the contact, and the resulting contraction of herpes, with its associated pain, satisfies the requirement of harm. Proving that transmission was intentional can be difficult, although the legal definition of intentional can be surprisingly broad and encompass situations in which the infected person had no desire to harm his or her sexual partner. While consent to intercourse would seem to be an invitation to contact, the consent does not extend to acquiring sexually transmitted infections. As in the case of negligence, full disclosure about one's genital herpes before engaging in intercourse is the best defense against charges of battery.

Misrepresentation is the third and least commonly applied basis for legal action in cases involving transmission of genital herpes. This situation involves the person with genital herpes making false representations (denying the illness or claiming not to be contagious) in order to induce a partner to engage in sexual activity. The partner relies on the misrepresentation in making a decision regarding intercourse and, as a result, suffers damage—in this case, medical expenses and the pain and suffering associated with acquiring genital herpes. The misrepresentation may either be a response to a direct inquiry or an unsolicited statement that one has no sexually transmissible diseases.

There are difficulties associated with bringing a successful lawsuit in connection with the transmission of genital herpes.

Because persons can be infected with the virus for years before they develop the signs and symptoms of disease, it can be very difficult to prove that the defendant and not some previous sexual partner was the cause of the plaintiff's infection. The only way to establish medically that a genital infection caused by herpes simplex virus type 2 was recently acquired is to conduct special tests to measure antibody against the type 2 virus with blood collected at the time of the first episode of disease. Since these tests are not part of the routine management of a patient with genital herpes they are rarely done. Hence, it is seldom possible to prove definitively how recently the infection was acquired. Indeed, even if the defendant has a history of genital herpes, it may be difficult to prove that he or she was the source of the virus causing genital herpes in the plaintiff. Where possible, the defendant's attorney will capitalize on this uncertainty and probe extensively into the plaintiff's prior sexual history, possibly establishing that the person had other, previous opportunities to become infected and suggesting to the jury that this individual may be a person of dubious morals. Such public scrutiny of one's private life can be a major deterrent to pursuing legal action.

With regard to causation, it is important to remember that most people with genital herpes are unaware that they have been infected, and therefore, unless they have a documented medical history of the disease, it may be very difficult to prove they were the source of the virus that infected a sexual partner. Another complicating factor may be the types of sexual acts in which people engage. For example, genital herpes due to the type 1 virus can result from oral-genital sex. Since most people are unaware that they may transmit or acquire genital herpes as a consequence of oral-genital sex, it may be difficult to establish negligence or misrepresentation. The defendant's attorney may consider a variety of strategies, including inter-spousal immunity (meaning that a husband or wife cannot

sue the other); the illegality of premarital or extramarital sexual relationships (damages cannot be recovered for an injury
that occurred during an illegal act); the concern that legal
action related to intimate relationships violates the person's
constitutional right to privacy; or the argument that, given
the prevalence of sexually transmitted diseases in our society,
anyone who fails to inquire about a partner's sexual health
or engages in unprotected sex is equally responsible for the
injury, especially if the relationship was brief (a so-called
one-night stand).

Some lawsuits in connection with the transmission of genital herpes have been successful. Punitive as well as compensa-
tory damages have been awarded in cases involving persons
who knew they had genital herpes, were aware of its contagious nature, and proceeded to have sexual contact without
disclosure. In 1996 there was a $600,000 judgment awarded
in connection with such a case. If a person does have recognizable genital herpes, a full disclosure of the illness before
engaging in sexual intercourse is the best strategy for protecting a partner from acquiring the infection and for avoiding a
possible lawsuit. Those contemplating filing a lawsuit should
have a frank discussion with their attorney regarding motiva-
tion in filing the suit and the potential personal difficulties that
they may encounter in pursuing an action in a public forum.

Health Insurance

Most people obtain health insurance through their place of
employment. This type of group health insurance generally
pays for routine medical visits and prescription drugs related
to genital herpes. Some even pay for counselling. Occasionally,
when someone changes jobs and thus insurance companies,

he or she may find that genital herpes is considered a preexisting condition. In this setting, the new insurer may exclude claims due to genital herpes for some defined period of time, or possibly bar coverage for the disease altogether. Such a situation can have significant financial consequences for the person taking daily antiviral prescription medication for a chronic condition. Problems associated with herpes and insurance are more likely to occur for those people with individual health insurance, policies designed for the self-employed and for those who work for small businesses. Some companies offering health insurance to individuals exclude coverage for genital herpes or deny coverage altogether for people with herpes. Within each state, an independent insurance agent should be able to identify companies and policies that will cover individuals with genital herpes. Those who have limited financial resources and are denied coverage for this disease might consider using local public health clinics if available. Such clinics often have extensive experience with people who have genital herpes and can frequently provide prescription medication for little or no cost.

8. Treating Herpes

Herpes simplex virus infections can be life threatening for some, including the newborn infant, the patient with a compromised immune system, or the individual with encephalitis. Because infections can be so dangerous in these special populations, they must be treated with potent prescription antiviral drugs given intravenously. The first episode of genital herpes, while not life threatening, can be severe (see chapter 4), and most people, if not all, who have this condition should be treated with prescription antiviral drugs taken by mouth. While there are prescription antiviral creams and ointments available, they are not as effective as drugs taken by mouth and should not be substituted for the more effective oral medications for first episode genital herpes. For the vast majority of people, recurrent genital and orolabial infections caused by herpes simplex virus are mild and self-limited, meaning that they heal eventually without treatment. Despite this situation, people seek treatment of these recurrent infections for a variety of reasons, including relief of pain or discomfort, because they find the herpetic sores cosmetically displeasing, and because they are concerned about transmitting the virus to others. In cases of recurrent genital or orolabial herpes, the goals of therapy can be either to reduce the severity and duration of the infection or to prevent it from recurring, possibly, in the process, reducing the likelihood that the individual will become contagious.

Several prescription antiviral drugs have been proven effective in treating and preventing recurrent genital herpes. Because recurrent herpes simplex virus infections are very common, people have also tried a variety of home remedies in an effort to control the illness. Most of these treatments have never been

carefully tested and some are potentially harmful. One diffi-
culty in assessing the effectiveness of therapies for herpes is the
placebo effect, a phenomenon whereby people perceive improvement in a medical condition when they are receiving a treatment
known to be ineffective, such as a sugar pill. A study done in
the 1960s showed that when doctors gave patients with recurrent herpes a placebo, about 3 out of 4 reported they had fewer
recurrences, and, if they did develop a recurrence, they believed
it to be less severe than when they were not on the "medicine."
This type of study shows that the power of suggestion (in this
case that a particular type of treatment is effective) can have a
profound influence on someone with herpes. While any relief,
real or perceived, is appreciated by those who suffer with herpes, people need to be aware that many or most home remedies, food supplements, and so-called cures for sale in magazines
and on the Internet are probably not effective and should not
be substituted for medications that have been shown to work.
The public should beware of claims that a treatment will cure
the latent infection. While there is ongoing scientific research
exploring how herpes simplex virus persists in nerve cells in its
latent state, as of this writing there is no treatment that has
been proven to rid the body of the virus once the latent infection has been established (see chapter 2). That means that all
currently available effective treatments control the disease, but
do not eliminate the infection. When people with genital herpes stop taking these medicines, the latent virus can reactivate
and cause recurrent infections.

Relief of Symptoms

Left alone, herpes sores eventually heal, and will do so faster
if they are kept clean and dry. Indeed, covering the lesions
with thick creams or ointments may actually cause the sores to

persist longer. Some people with genital herpes find that warm baths with or without Epsom salts or baking soda added to the water provide some relief. Patients are usually advised to wear loose cotton underclothing so as to avoid rubbing or irritating the sores. Steroid creams available without prescription in pharmacies and supermarkets should not be used in treating herpes lesions. These creams can interfere with the action of the body's immune system in the skin and actually worsen the disease, slowing down the healing process and allowing the infection to spread. For some, nonprescription pain medication like aspirin, acetaminophen, or ibuprofen can alleviate the pain and discomfort caused by the sores. Those who experience significant pain with their illness should talk to their doctors about prescription pain medications.

The Stress Connection

Many people who experience orolabial or genital herpes report that their recurrences can be brought on by stress. While there is little scientific evidence to support this belief, stress reduction is desirable for many reasons, even if it is never shown to be of benefit in controlling herpes outbreaks. Desirable habits that may reduce or help a person cope with stress include adequate sleep, a well-balanced diet, avoidance of tobacco and recreational drugs, and regular participation in an exercise program. Methods for managing stress include meditation, hypnosis, biofeedback, visualization, and psychotherapy. People who feel that stress is a major contributor to their herpes outbreaks should discuss stress management programs with a health care provider. Insurance policies may include coverage for some of these programs.

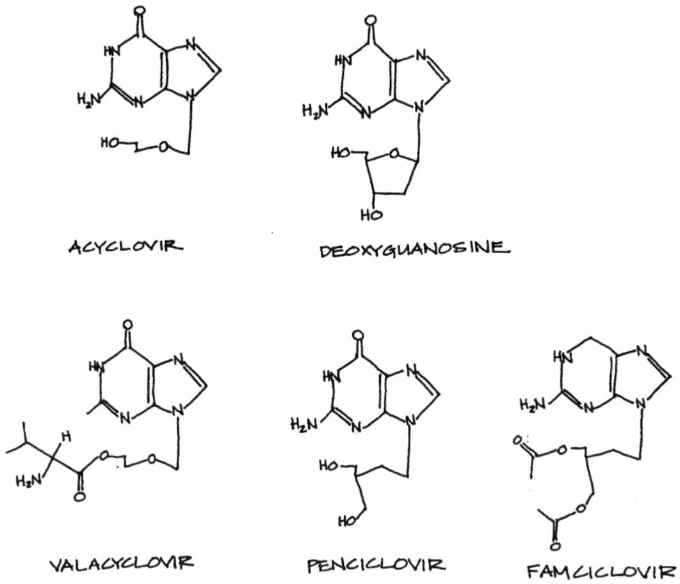

Figure 8.1 Structures of four drugs plus deoxyguanosine

Prescription Antiviral Drugs

Currently in the United States there are four prescription drugs that are used routinely in the treatment of herpes simplex virus infections of the skin: acyclovir, valacyclovir, penciclovir, and famciclovir. Valacyclovir and famciclovir are *prodrugs*, medicines that are designed to break down in the body to an active form—in this case, acyclovir and penciclovir, respectively. These medicines belong to the class of antiviral drugs called *nucleoside analogs*, a term which refers to the fact that their chemical structures are similar to nucleosides, the building blocks of ribonucleic acid (RNA) and deoxyribonucleic acid (DNA) (fig. 8.1).

These drugs act by interfering with virus replication. They have little or no effect on normal cells, but in virus-infected cells they are activated to a form that can block the virus's ability to make copies of itself (see chapter 2). This limits the spread of the infection and makes it easier for the body's defense systems to control the infection.

Acyclovir has been available in the United States since the mid-1980s. It has an excellent safety record and has been used by hundreds of thousands of people for the management of herpes simplex virus infections. It is available as an ointment for topical use, in liquid, capsule, and tablet form to be taken by mouth, and in a sterile solution for intravenous administration. The oral form is much more effective than the topical form for treating herpes infections of the skin. Because of its pharmacological properties, oral acyclovir must be taken 3 to 5 times daily, depending on whether the drug is being used for first episode or recurrent genital herpes. Within the infected cell, the virus converts acyclovir to an active form that is incorporated into a replicating strand of viral DNA, halting its synthesis. Thus, acyclovir is referred to as a *chain terminator*. Acyclovir and related drugs work only on actively replicating herpes simplex virus and have no effect on the latent, nonreplicating virus that resides within neurons. For that reason, acyclovir treatment does not eradicate the latent infection.

Some herpes simplex viruses have developed resistance to acyclovir, meaning that the drug no longer blocks the replication of the virus. In most cases, the resistance is due to subtle changes in the structure of the viral protein that converts acyclovir to the active form of the drug. Acyclovir is not effective in treating infections caused by such viruses. Fortunately, acyclovir-resistant herpes simplex viruses are rare; they are seen almost exclusively in people with impaired immune systems. Infections caused by acyclovir-resistant viruses can be treated with other antiviral drugs that do not require the viral protein for conversion to their active form. Examples include foscarnet and cidofovir, which also act by blocking viral DNA synthesis. While having many side effects, these alternative drugs can be useful. A patient who has been using acyclovir for the control of his or her recurrent herpes and feels that the drug is no longer working should discuss this concern with a physician or other health care provider. Generally there is usually some simple explanation for the decreased effectiveness, such as a change in intestinal absorption. Some fear that after taking acyclovir or any antiviral drug for several years their bodies will develop a "tolerance" to the medication, so that it will no longer be of use. There is no scientific evidence that acyclovir's effectiveness decreases over a prolonged period of time; many people have used it daily for years and found no change. In the United States acyclovir is marketed by the GlaxoSmithKline Company under the trade name Zovirax®. Several companies produce generic acyclovir.

Valacyclovir is a chemically modified form of acyclovir that allows more of the drug to be absorbed from the stomach and intestine into the bloodstream; that is, it has a greater *bioavailability* than acyclovir. After absorption from the gastrointestinal tract, valacyclovir is rapidly converted to acyclovir. Valacyclovir appears to be just as effective as acyclovir in treating genital herpes and has the advantage that it need be taken only once or twice daily. An oral form of valacyclovir is being marketed in the United States by the GlaxoSmithKline Company under the trade name Valtrex®.

Penciclovir is an antiviral drug that is closely related to acyclovir and acts in the same way to inhibit virus replication. Because penciclovir is poorly absorbed from the gastrointestinal tract, there is no oral form of the drug. There is, however, a cream form for topical use in the treatment of recurrent fever blisters (herpes labialis). The penciclovir product is the first topical drug to be proven effective in the treatment of fever blisters. To get around the problem of poor absorption, a prodrug, *famciclovir*, was developed; it has good bioavailability and is rapidly converted to penciclovir after it reaches the bloodstream. It has an excellent safety profile and rarely has any side effects. Famciclovir has been shown to be effective in the treatment of primary and recurrent genital herpes when given 2 or 3 times daily. Most acyclovir-resistant strains of herpes simplex virus are also resistant to penciclovir; for that reason, famciclovir should not be used to treat such infections. Penciclovir (Denavir®) and famciclovir (Famvir®) are sold in the United States by Novartis.

Treatment Versus Suppression

Antiviral drugs work with the body's immune system to help control viral infections. Viruses can cause injury that may take days or weeks to heal after the virus has been eliminated from the body. Thus, even if a drug is very effective at stopping the virus from multiplying, a person taking it is likely to have signs and symptoms of the illness for many days after he or she starts taking the drug. The way to get the best results from antiviral drug therapy is to begin treatment as soon as possible—the longer the delay is, the less effective the drug will be. Because early treatment is important, many doctors will give prescriptions that their patients with recurrent herpes can keep at home and begin to use at the first signs of an outbreak. This is referred to as *patient-initiated therapy*.

Because herpes outbreaks are by and large unpredictable, some people prefer to take antiviral drugs on a daily basis in anticipation of an outbreak. Prescription antiviral drugs taken daily can prevent recurrent infections; such treatment is referred to as *suppressive therapy*. It is uncertain whether daily treatment acts to prevent the virus from reactivating in the ganglia (see chapter 2) or simply blocks its replication in skin cells. However it works, suppressive therapy can prevent or significantly reduce the number and severity of recognized outbreaks of recurrent genital herpes. It can also reduce asymptomatic virus shedding. Suppressive therapy with valacyclovir has been proven to reduce the likelihood of transmission of genital herpes. It should be emphasized that some people on suppressive therapy do experience breakthroughs and that transmission of virus from individuals on suppressive therapy to their sexual partners does occur. The reasons for these failures are uncertain, but one likely explanation is that the person has missed taking a dose; in such a case, sufficient time may pass for the recurrence to begin before the next dose is taken. Theoretically, if a person taking a long-acting antiviral drug once daily misses a dose, as much as 48 hours could pass before the next one, ample time for the virus to reactivate or initiate replication in skin cells.

Treatment of First Episode Genital Herpes

All cases of first episode genital herpes should probably be treated. The first episode is typically more severe than the recurrent infections, and people experiencing the first episode of genital herpes are more likely to have complications (see chapter 4). Acyclovir, valacyclovir, and famciclovir taken by mouth have all been shown to be effective in treating first-episode genital herpes. People taking these drugs have a shorter, less painful illness. Regrettably, people who receive treatment for their first episode of genital herpes later have recurrent infections just as do those who receive no treatment. This finding indicates that treatment during the first infection does not interfere with the establishment of latent infection.

Episodic Treatment of Recurrent Genital Herpes

Most people with genital infection caused by herpes simplex virus type 2 will experience recurrent infections. Very short courses of antiviral therapy (one day of famciclovir, two days of acyclovir, or three days of valacyclovir) have been shown to shorten the overall duration of an outbreak of recurrent genital herpes up to three days. As discussed above, treatment is most effective when begun early, ideally during the prodromal phase before any skin lesions begin to develop. Patients who experience frequent or severe recurrences or have significant emotional difficulties caused by the recurrent infection should consider suppressive therapy instead of episodic treatment of the recurrences. Topical acyclovir treatment is not effective in reducing the signs and symptoms that accompany recurrent infections and should not be substituted for effective treatment with drugs taken by mouth.

Suppression of Recurrent Genital Herpes

Genital herpes, like high blood pressure or diabetes, is a chronic illness. Suppression therapy for genital herpes, like insulin therapy for diabetes, does not cure the illness but does control it. Daily suppressive therapy with acyclovir, valacyclovir, or famciclovir is very effective in reducing the frequency of recognized recurrent infections and asymptomatic virus shedding. Daily treatment of the infected person with

1 gram of valacyclovir has been shown to cut the risk in half of transmitting genital herpes to a sexual partner. Condoms have also been proven to lower but not eliminate the risk of spreading genital herpes. The best strategy for reducing the likelihood of transmission of the virus is probably the combination of daily suppressive therapy and condom use. Suppressive therapy should be considered for anyone who has frequent or severe outbreaks of genital herpes or for those who are particularly troubled by recurrent infections. Typically the drug is taken daily for one year, at which time the patient and his or her medical provider discuss discontinuing it. If there are persistent concerns regarding recurrent infections, the drug is usually continued; otherwise, it is stopped, and healthcare provider and patient wait to see whether new recurrences develop, and, if so, how severe they are. If problems arise, the patient should be started again on suppressive therapy. The safety and effectiveness of daily suppressive therapy has been established in people taking the medications for many years.

The Pregnant Woman

None of the currently available drugs effective in treating herpes simplex virus infections are approved by the Food and Drug Administration for use by pregnant women. They are all probably effective in treating genital herpes during pregnancy, but their safety has not been studied. Because they interfere with DNA synthesis, they all pose a theoretical risk to the developing fetus, but so does the mother's herpes simplex virus infection. Healthcare professionals caring for the pregnant woman with genital herpes must carefully weigh the potential risks and benefits of treatment. In general, pregnant women experiencing a severe first episode of genital herpes will be prescribed antiviral therapy, while those with mild, recurrent infections are not treated. Some women on suppressive acyclovir do not discover that they are pregnant until several weeks into the pregnancy. So far, babies born to women who were taking acyclovir early in pregnancy don't appear more likely to have developmental problems. However, women on daily suppressive therapy should stop taking the medicine while pregnant and remain off it while they are breast-feeding.

The American College of Obstetrics and Gynecology advocates using chronic suppressive anti-herpes therapy for the last four weeks of pregnancy in women who have a history of recurrent genital herpes or who developed the first episode of the disease during the pregnancy, in order to reduce the need for cesarean deliveries and decrease the likelihood that the virus will spread to the baby (see chapter 6).

Over-the-Counter Drugs, Nutritional Supplements, and Home Remedies

Because herpes infections are so common, people have tried all sorts of different remedies to treat or prevent this ailment. Unfortunately, few nonprescription remedies have been carefully tested, and support for their use usually comes from testimonials about their effectiveness. Since herpes outbreaks occur unpredictably and with varying degrees of severity, determining a treatment's effectiveness is difficult without carefully comparing it to another one known to be ineffective. Such studies are called double-blind, placebo-controlled trials because neither the patient nor the healthcare provider knows whether the patient is receiving the study drug (the home remedy) or a sugar pill (the placebo). Because people can be fooled about the effectiveness of treatments for herpes, it is important that those considering a home remedy avoid any treatment that might make the condition worse (delay healing or spread the infection); neither should they discontinue prescription medicine that has been proven to be effective in favor of treatments that have not.

People have tried a variety of over-the-counter medicines intended for other uses in an attempt to find convenient products that offer some relief from the pain and discomfort of herpes. Products that contain xylocaine or phenol (for example, Campho-Phenique®) numb the area temporarily, giving pain relief but having no real effect on the infection. Steroid creams like Cortaid® can make the sores less painful, but they delay healing and, because they interfere with the ability of the immune system to work effectively in the treated skin, can actually help the infection spread; they can also increase the risk of yeast infections. Oral antibiotics like ampicillin or sulfa-containing compounds have no effect on the herpes virus and can also increase the risk of yeast infection. Topical/intravaginal preparations for the treatment of yeast infections not only are ineffective against herpes, but, if applied directly to the sores, can slow healing and prolong the illness. Some people try anti-inflammatory drugs like Motrin® (ibuprofen). Placebo-controlled trials showed that ibuprofen taken daily did not prevent recurrent infections, nor did it reduce the severity of the recurrences. Nonoxynol-9, the detergent in many spermicides, is known to inactivate herpes simplex virus in the test tube, but it is ineffective in the treatment of recurrent herpes infections. Cimetidine (Tagamet®), which is used in treating duodenal ulcers, has been shown to be ineffective in preventing recurrent genital herpes.

People have also tried products purchased from chemical supply companies. Some chemicals like ether, chloroform, or iodine solutions can inactivate the virus in the skin when applied topically, but have no effect on the pain and discomfort caused by the sores and can irritate the skin, causing the sores to heal more slowly. Butylated hydroxytoluene (BHT), a phenolic antioxidant food preservative, is not effective in treating herpes and has been known to cause serious stomach disorders as well as cancer in animals given large doses. A sugar related to glucose, 2-deoxy-D-glucose (2DG), has antiviral activity in the test tube but is not effective in the treatment of recurrent herpes infections.

Attempts to enhance the immune system have been made in the hope that fewer or less severe outbreaks would be the result. For many years the smallpox vaccine was used for this purpose; however, it was not effective and occasionally caused severe or life-threatening reactions. Fortunately, the vaccine is no longer available for this use. Other vaccines, including those for polio and flu, have also been used for the treatment of recurrent herpes; again, they have not been shown to be effective. Therapeutic herpes vaccines (Lupidon) are available in parts of Europe, but their effectiveness has not been conclusively proven. As discussed in the next chapter, therapeutic vaccines are still being investigated and may someday be useful in controlling recurrent herpes infections. For the time being, however, no vaccines are available for the prevention or treatment of herpes.

Nutritional supplements have been advocated by some as a "cure" for herpes. There are those who believe that a conspiracy of physicians and large pharmaceutical companies is suppressing information about such products, but, in fact, no data exist establishing the effectiveness of any nutritional supplement in the prevention or treatment of herpes simplex virus infections. Testimonials have been given, but since, as we have seen, people can perceive benefit even from sugar pills, one should be very skeptical about any treatment that has not been carefully tested. (What do we mean by "carefully tested"? For approval by the U.S. Food and Drug Administration, a herpes treatment must be studied in a controlled clinical trial in which some people get the new treatment and others get an ineffective medicine, or placebo. The patients do not know which they are receiving, nor does the healthcare provider. Above all, the new treatment must be proven safe; it must also be more effective than the placebo in preventing outbreaks or in reducing the duration or severity of symptoms.) Supplements that have been used by people with herpes include zinc, vitamins B_{12}, C, and E, red algae, various herbs, and lysine (an amino acid used mostly as an animal feed supplement). There being no proof that any of these (or any other) "natural" treatments work, people who choose such therapies should consider the following points: (1) Is the treatment safe? Beware of using very large doses (megadoses) of any product, because small amounts of impurities may cause significant problems when ingested in large quantities; (2) What is the cost of the therapy? Are you spending more on unproven treatment than you would on prescription drugs that are known to be effective? (3) Is there someone you can complain to if the therapy doesn't work or makes you sick? Be skeptical of remedies advertised in newspapers, magazines, or on the Internet and sold via the mail. These companies tend to disappear after they have received your money and sometimes before they have sent you any product.

With regard to any unproven product, the consumer must always remember the Latin warning *caveat emptor*—let the buyer beware. With regard to products promised as cures and sold by unknown companies through the mail, the consumer should remember the statement attributed to P. T. Barnum: "There's a sucker born every minute."

9. The Search for Vaccines and Microbicides

Vaccines protect people against infectious diseases. When a person becomes infected with a disease-causing microorganism, the body's immune system produces a variety of defensive responses that kill the microbe. Vaccines cause the body to produce these same disease-fighting responses without the person actually getting the infection. After immunization with a vaccine, the body has the defenses ready, so if the person is exposed to the disease-causing organism, the immune system can act quickly to destroy the invading microbe before it causes disease. For maximum effectiveness, the immune system makes responses that are tailored to each specific microbe; similarly, vaccines are designed to protect against specific disease-causing organisms. In other words, no single vaccine protects against all infections; instead, a series of vaccines protects against a series of illnesses.

Scientists have developed several ways to make vaccines. Some vaccines consist of *attenuated living organisms*, in which the whole microbe has been weakened (attenuated) so that it cannot cause disease but can induce the immune system to make protective responses. Because they replicate in the body, the organisms in live-attenuated vaccines cause the immune system to respond as it does to the disease-causing organisms; this includes humoral (antibody) and cellular responses (see chapter 2). Examples of live, attenuated vaccines include the oral polio and the chickenpox vaccines. Vaccines may also consist of killed organisms, which are incapable of causing disease. Some vaccines containing killed or *inactivated* organisms, like the inactivated polio vaccine, can be very effective; others, however, are ineffective, and some actually induce undesirable immune responses, as was the case with inactivated vaccines for measles, respiratory syncytial virus, and chlamydia. The reasons why these vaccines fail are complex but probably relate to changes in the structure of the organism that occur as a consequence of the inactivation process and to differences in how the immune system "sees" replicating organisms compared with dead ones. Inactivated vaccines are very good at inducing the immune system to make antibodies against the organism, but they are less effective in inducing cellular immune responses. This means that the protective responses are less broad and in some cases less durable. To improve on the protective effect of inactivated vaccines, scientists have developed adjuvants, chemicals that enhance the *immunogenicity* of the vaccine. Immunogenicity refers to the ability of a vaccine to induce strong and long-lasting humoral and cellular immune responses. Adjuvants may cause an inactivated vaccine to induce greater cellular immune responses and may lengthen the time before a booster dose is needed. Unfortunately, adjuvants can also increase the *reactogenicity* of the vaccine, which is the ability of a vaccine to cause undesirable reactions such as pain at the site of injection, headache, muscle ache, or fever. Adjuvants that are the most potent at enhancing vaccine immunogenicity tend to be the most reactogenic. The development of certain types of new vaccines is limited because of the reactogenicity of potentially useful adjuvants.

Breakthroughs in biotechnology have allowed for the development of four modern approaches to making vaccines. *Subunit vaccines* consist of small pieces, or subunits, of the microbe, usually protein components of the outer structure of the organism. These pieces tend to be the part of the organism first seen by the immune system and are selected because they are highly immunogenic, especially with regard to the magnitude of the antibody response they can induce. Because they cannot replicate, they generally do not induce good cellular immune responses unless combined with adjuvants. Recently developed vaccines against hepatitis B virus are an example of a subunit vaccine. *Replication-impaired viral vaccines* consist of viruses that have been genetically engineered so that they can only undergo a single round of replication. These vaccine viruses cannot produce progeny virus and hence are incapable of causing typical viral disease. Because they go through one round of replication, they can induce both antibody and cellular immune responses. No replication-impaired vaccines are currently licensed by the Food and Drug Administration, although some are currently being tested in clinical trials. *Live-vectored vaccines* refer to attenuated viruses that have been engineered so as to carry a small piece of foreign DNA or RNA that encodes for an immunogenic protein. Vector refers to the attenuated virus that carries the foreign gene. An example that has been studied in people is the smallpox vaccine (vaccinia virus), engineered to contain the gene that encodes for the gp160 protein of the human immunodeficiency virus. A person immunized with the live vector makes immune responses both to the vector and to the product of the extra gene. This type of vaccine should induce both antibody and cellular immune responses, but because it only contains one or two foreign genes, the responses are narrowly directed to a limited number of possible immunogenic proteins. *Nucleic acid-based vaccines*, sometimes referred to as naked DNA vaccines, are a very new development. Scientists have shown that injection into skin or muscle of small pieces of DNA or RNA that encode immunogenic proteins results in the production of antibody and cell-mediated immune responses directed against the protein. Apparently the RNA or DNA is taken up by cells through an unknown mechanism where it is used to make copies of the protein it encodes. This protein then induces the immune system to make the types of responses usually produced by replicating organisms. Several nucleic acid vaccines are being clinically tested to determine if they are safe and effective.

Goals for a Herpes Simplex Virus Vaccine

Infection occurs when a microorganism replicates in the host. The replicating microbe can cause disease that is manifested by recognizable signs and symptoms of illness, or the infection may have no obvious signs of illness, in which case it is said to be asymptomatic. In the best of all possible worlds, a vaccine against herpes would induce "sterilizing immunity," which would completely protect the oral or genital tract and associated sensory ganglia from becoming infected. When exposed to the virus, the immunized person's vaccine-induced immune responses would prevent the virus from replicating; hence, the host would become neither ill nor latently infected. What, in fact, vaccines do is change the person's susceptibility to infection and protect them against developing disease. After being immunized a person must be exposed to higher amounts of the disease-causing microbe before the infection can get started. Even then, the infection is much more likely to be asymptomatic; in other words the person does not become sick. *This is an important concept: most vaccines prevent disease but do not prevent infection.* Studies have shown that, when an animal is exposed to herpes simplex virus for the first time, the virus replicates in the genital tract and spreads to the ganglia, and the animal develops an illness similar to genital herpes in humans. If the animal is reexposed to a different strain of herpes simplex virus after recovery from the first episode of genital herpes, the new strain of virus replicates in the genital tract but does not spread to the ganglia, and the animal does not develop any signs of genital herpes. In this setting, the immune responses produced by the first infection did not protect the animal against reinfection (although it required 100 times more virus to cause the infection) but did protect against spread of the virus beyond the genital tract and prevented the animal from developing a symptomatic illness. Theoretically it should be possible for a vaccine to provide the same protection that "natural" infection does. Therefore, a realistic goal might be the development of a vaccine which, while not preventing virus replication at the portal of entry (the skin), does prevent establishment of latent infection in sensory ganglia and signs and symptoms of genital herpes. In this setting, exposure would result in an asymptomatic infection, but since no latent infection was established, the person would not have recurrent infections.

A less ambitious but definitely feasible goal would be the development of a vaccine that provides partial protection against symptomatic genital herpes. This goal is supported by clinical studies of a subunit vaccine that is discussed later in this chapter. It is possible that a partially effective vaccine might have considerable public health impact by decreasing the susceptibility of uninfected people and the potential for transmission in those vaccinated people who become infected.

With all these theoretical considerations in mind, a special committee of experts empaneled by the prestigious National Academy of Sciences suggested that a successful herpes simplex virus vaccine should provide a 50 percent reduction in the number of symptomatic primary infections, a 75 percent reduction in the number of recurrences, and approximately a 60 percent reduction in the severity of disease.

Vaccines Containing Live Virus or Replication—Impaired Viruses

Live virus vaccines are generally produced by the repetitive growing of a virulent virus in cells in a test tube until some change occurs making the virus attenuated (crippled), so that it is still immunogenic but now incapable of causing disease. This strategy has worked for polio and varicella-zoster (chicken pox), but has not been successful for herpes simplex virus, which has a nasty tendency to revert unpredictably to a virulent, disease-causing virus. There are also concerns regarding the ability of a live virus to establish a latent infection and potentially to reactivate. Another approach that addresses the stability issue is the use of molecular genetic methods to engineer stably attenuated viruses. This strategy has been successfully used to develop veterinary vaccines for pseudorabies virus, one closely related to herpes simplex virus. Bernard Roizman at the University of Chicago further extended this approach by engineering attenuated intertypic viruses that were part type 1 and part type 2. In theory, these engineered virus vaccines should protect against infection caused by either the type 1 or the type 2 virus. One of Dr. Roizman's engineered viruses, R7020, was shown to be safe and effective in animals, but when it was tested by the Institut Merieux in French college students was found to be overly attenuated and poorly immunogenic. Based on this experience and the identification of additional virulence genes, Dr. Roizman and his collaborators have engineered new intertypic mutants which are being further developed by Medimmune, Inc.

A novel variation on genetically attenuated viruses was the development of replication-impaired viruses. This approach to making a herpes simplex virus vaccine was developed independently by Tony Minson at Cambridge University and David Knipe at Harvard University. The idea was to delete a gene that is essential for virus replication but then to grow the defective virus in a genetically engineered cell line that expresses the missing viral gene product. The resulting virus is capable of infecting normal cells but cannot make the missing gene product and thus cannot replicate; hence, it is limited to a single infectious cycle without spread of infection to other cells. Studies have shown these viruses to be safe and effective in animals. Dr. Minson's approach was developed by a British biotech firm, Cantab Pharmaceuticals (now Celtic Pharma) and their vaccine called TA-HSV Disc was shown to be safe and immunogenic in humans.

An approach that retains some of the immunological advantages of a live virus vaccine while avoiding concerns regarding herpes attenuation is the use of live virus vectors. In this approach a herpes simplex virus gene(s) encoding an immunogenic protein(s) is inserted into a replication-competent virus vector. When immunized with the vector, the host makes humoral (antibody) and cellular immune responses to the proteins encoded by the vector, including the herpes protein(s). A number of vectors have been proposed, including vaccinia, adenovirus, poliovirus, rhinoviruses, and canarypox. Studies have shown that live viral vectors encoding herpes genes are safe and immunogenic in animals. An interesting example of the live viral vector is a virus developed by Jeff Cohen and his colleagues at the National Institutes of Health. They engineered the licensed, live, attenuated Oka varicella-zoster (chicken pox) vaccine to contain the gD gene of herpes simplex virus type 2. They showed that guinea pigs immunized with the modified chicken pox vaccine made antibody to the herpes gD protein and were partially protected against experimental genital herpes infection. The use of live viral vectors warrants further study, although currently there are no live vectored herpes vaccines in clinical trials.

Vaccines Containing Killed Virus

Vaccines made by completely inactivating the virus have a potential safety advantage over live virus vaccines, since the killed virus cannot replicate or cause infection. However, they have the disadvantage of perhaps inducing less broad and less durable immune responses than live virus vaccines. Killed herpes vaccines have a long and unsuccessful history. In the 1930s, vaccines were made by infecting guinea pigs or rabbits with herpes simplex virus; the infected tissues were ground up, chemicals were added to inactivate the virus, and the mixture was homogenized before it was injected into volunteers. In the 1950s, vaccines were prepared by using ultraviolet radiation to inactivate virus grown in developing chicken eggs, a method still used to make some flu vaccines. By the 1960s, virus was being grown in test tubes containing cells and inactivated by ultraviolet irradiation, formalin treatment, or heat. These early vaccines were largely tested in open clinical trials, meaning that all the volunteers received the vaccine, with no group of nonimmunized subjects for comparison purposes.

One inactivated vaccine developed by the Eli Lilly Co. was evaluated in a careful double-blind, placebo-controlled trial to determine its effectiveness in reducing recurrent herpes infections. The study found that 70 percent of the vaccine recipients thought they were having fewer recurrences, while 76 percent of the people receiving the ineffective placebo believed the same thing about themselves! This study illustrates the importance of study design in testing herpes vaccines and points out how the power of suggestion can influence one's perception of a chronic illness.

Several killed vaccines were developed in the 1970s and 1980s. Lupidon H (from the type 1 virus) and Lupidon G (from the type 2 virus) are heat-inactivated preparations made from virus grown in developing chicken eggs. The vaccines are produced by the Hermal Boots Company in Germany. They are used as therapeutic vaccines (for the treatment of recurrent herpes), but there is limited data indicating that they work. The Dundarov vaccine is manufactured in Bulgaria and contains chemically inactivated whole virus (type 1, type 2, or both). Like Lupidon, this vaccine is intended for therapeutic use but also lacks proof of effectiveness. The Skinner vaccine was developed in England and consists of a chemically treated, detergent extract of type 1 virus grown in human cells. It has been tested as both a prophylactic (preventive) and a therapeutic vaccine, although its effectiveness for either use has never been clearly proven. The Cappel vaccine, developed in Belgium, is also intended for both therapeutic and prophylactic use. It is a DNA-free virion envelope vaccine made by detergent disruption of type 2 virus grown in cells followed by ultracentrifugation to separate the virion envelope proteins from other materials. The vaccine has been shown to be immunogenic, but its effectiveness has not been tested in controlled trials. The Kutinova vaccine, prepared by Czech investigators, is made of type 1 viral glycoproteins adsorbed to aluminum hydroxide (alum). It was designed for therapeutic use. Limited clinical trials suggest that the vaccine is neither immunogenic nor effective. A recent entry into the realm of killed vaccines was a viral glycoprotein product made by Merck and Company in the United States. It was similar to the Kutinova vaccine except that it was prepared from type 2 virus. Initial clinical testing showed that the vaccine induced virus-specific immune responses. Unfortunately, a large, well-designed clinical trial showed the vaccine was not effective in preventing genital herpes. This failure may have been partly due to the fact that the vaccine was poorly immunogenic at the dose tested.

Genetically Engineered Subunit Vaccines

The advent of genetic engineering, a method by which cells can be genetically altered to make new products, allowed the manufacture of large quantities of immunogenic proteins without the need to work with virus-infected cells. From a vaccine perspective, this approach has the safety advantage of ensuring that the preparation is free of infectious virus or viral DNA. Subunit vaccines, however, have some shortcomings. Since they contain only a fraction of the antigens present in a whole virus, the subunit vaccine can only induce immune responses to a limited number of possible immunogens. Also, like killed vaccines, subunit vaccines generally induce a less durable and less broad immune response; purified proteins alone tend not to induce a full array of cell-mediated responses. To address this problem, purified protein(s) have been formulated with adjuvants.

Subunit herpes simplex virus vaccine development has largely focused on two envelope glycoproteins, gB and gD.

These are major viral proteins recognized by the immune system with regard to antibody production, but it is uncertain whether they are the predominant viral target for cell-mediated responses. These recombinant glycoprotein vaccines have been shown in animal studies to be immunogenic and protective. Four subunit vaccine preparations have been evaluated in clinical studies. A vaccine developed by the Chiron Corporation containing recombinant truncated type 2 gD adsorbed to alum was tested as a therapeutic vaccine for the control of frequent recurrent genital herpes. The vaccine was found to be both immunogenic and modestly effective. A second vaccine was prepared by adding MF59, an immunopotentiating emulsion, to the original Chiron vaccine. The immunogenicity of this formulation was disappointing; it was reported to induce a high frequency of local reactions at the site of injection, and was found to be ineffective in reducing recurrent genital herpes. Chiron also developed a vaccine containing recombinant type 2 gB and gD with MF59 that was intended for prophylactic use. Initial trials indicated the vaccine was immunogenic. However, clinical evaluation of the vaccine was halted in late 1996 when the company announced that the vaccine had failed to protect recipients from type 2 genital infection. The fourth subunit vaccine tested in humans was developed by SmithKline Beecham Biologicals (now GlaxoSmithKline Biologicals) in Belgium. It contains a recombinant type 2 gD and alum combined with the potent adjuvant 3dMPL. The vaccine is well tolerated and induces humoral and cellular immune responses superior to those produced by gD/alum alone. The GlaxoSmithKline vaccine was tested in over 3,000 volunteers and was shown to protect some women but to be ineffective in men. The reason for this sex difference is unknown but some protection in women is an exciting discovery. The company and the U.S. National Institutes of

Health are currently conducting a trial of the vaccine in healthy young women. The study is called the HERPEVAC trial.

Nucleic Acid Vaccines

The development of nucleic acid-based vaccines has provided a new strategy for controlling herpes infections. Vaccines consisting of small pieces of viral DNA encoding type 1 or type 2 glycoproteins have been shown to induce humoral and cellular immune responses and to protect mice and guinea pigs against herpes simplex virus challenge. This is a burgeoning field with many large and small companies exploring its potential. In the United States, Vical, Inc., and Merck are involved in the preclinical development of DNA-based vaccines for the prevention of herpes simplex virus infections. An American biotech company, Apollon, Inc., has already begun clinical testing in humans.

The Future for Vaccines

Despite setbacks, the involvement of many talented investigators and of large and successful vaccine companies suggests that within a few years there should be a vaccine available to help reduce a person's risk of acquiring genital herpes (and other types of herpes simplex virus infections as well). Even if we succeed only in making a modestly effective vaccine, it is likely that many people will benefit. With regard to the development of vaccines for treating genital herpes, the verdict is not yet in as to whether such products will be superior to currently available antiviral drug therapy. Despite the uncertainty, researchers continue to examine how vaccines might be used to benefit people already infected with the herpes virus.

Microbicides

Microbicides are a new approach to protecting people against sexually transmitted infections including HIV and genital herpes. These products are intended to be used in the vagina or rectum before (and possibly shortly after) sexual intercourse. They might actually destroy the microbe before it can cause infection or they could prevent the microbe from attaching to cells, which is necessary for viral infection. Some possible microbicides actually increase the effectiveness of local immunities, making the person more resistant to the infection. Different types of formulation are also being tested, including gels, suppositories, and films. Several organizations and companies are currently involved in microbicide research and development, including the Population Council (Carraguard®), Starpharma (VivaGel®), Indevus Pharmaceuticals (Pro 2000), ReProtect (BufferGel), Gilead (Tenofovir/PMPAgel), and Biosyn, Inc. (Saavy®). This is a very exciting strategy and one that can be female-controlled, which is not always the case for condoms. It is hoped that within the next few years microbicides will be available. Depending on how they work, these products could be used by uninfected women to protect themselves from getting infected or by infected women to reduce the likelihood that they would spread their infection to a susceptible sexual partner.

Appendix A

Local Support Groups

The Herpes Resource Center of the nonprofit American Social Health Association has an affiliated network of local support groups called HELP groups. These provide a safe, confidential environment where people can get accurate information and share experiences, fears, and feelings with others who are also concerned about herpes. Local groups come and go, so if you cannot locate one in your area, inquire further at the Herpes Resource Center at (919) 361–8485 or HRC, P.O. Box 13827, Research Triangle Park, NC 27709.

ARIZONA
Phoenix Valley HELP
Phoenix, AZ
(602) 867-6613
E-mail: PHXVHG@hotmail.com
Web: http://www.valleyhelpgroup.com

CALIFORNIA
Los Angeles HELP
Culver City, CA
(310) 281-7511
E-mail: info@lahelp.org
Web: http://www.lahelp.org

Orange County HELP
Orange, CA
(949) 753-2580
Web: http://www.lahelp.org/index2.htm

San Diego City HELP
San Diego, CA
(619) 491-1194
E-mail: Questions@SanDiegoCityHelp.org
Web: http://www.SanDiegoCityHELP.org

San Francisco HELP
San Francisco, CA
(650) 704-4021
E-mail: HELP_SF@yahoo.com

CONNECTICUT
Manchester HELP
Manchester, CT
(860) 445-5863 (Annie)
(860) 666-0075 (Susan)
E-mail: hsv2secret@aol.com

DELAWARE
HELP of Delaware
c/o Omega Medical Center
Newark, DE
(302) 368-9625

DISTRICT OF COLUMBIA
HELP of Washington
Washington, DC
(301) 369-1323
Web: http://www.herpeshelpofwashington.org

FLORIDA
Broward and Palm Beach HELP
Coral Springs, FL
(954) 896-9788
E-mail: helpinsfl@yahoo.com

Central Florida HELP
Orlando, FL
(407) 263-5347
Web: http://www.geocities.com/orlandohelpgroup

Tampa Bay HELP
2 Groups—Tampa and Clearwater
(813) 677-1633

Jacksonville HELP
Jacksonville, FL
(877) 221-7896
E-mail: jacksonvillehelp@yahoo.com
Web: http://www.jacksonvillehelp.org

GEORGIA
Atlanta HELP
Atlanta, GA
(404) 294-6364

ILLINOIS
Chicago HELP
Chicago, IL
(773) 660-0416
E-mail: info@chicagohelp.org
Web: http://www.chicagohelp.org

INDIANA
Indy HELP
Indianapolis, IN
(317) 221-8313
E-mail: IndyHelp@yahoo.com
Web: http://www.indyhelp.com

Southern Indiana HELP
Shirley, IN
(765) 785-9219
E-mail: gayla@hrtc.net

LOUISIANA
New Orleans HELP
P.O. Box 55811
Metarie, LA 70055
(504) 568-2937
E-mail: nohg@rtconline.com

MAINE
Maine HELP
c/o City of Bangor STD Clinic
Bangor, ME
(207) 947-0700

MASSACHUSETTS
Boston HELP
Boston, MA
(781) 648-4266
Web: http://www.bostonherpes.org

MICHIGAN
Metro Detroit HELP
Eastpointe, MI
(586) 447-2699
E-mail: info@metrodetroithelp.org
Web: http://www.metrodetroithelp.org

Traverse City HELP
Traverse City, MI
(800) 442-7315 (toll-free)
E-mail: monkey_method@hotmail.com

Washtenaw County HELP
Novi, MI
(248) 788-5816
E-mail: wchfacilitator@aol.com
Web: http://www.annarborhelp.org

MINNESOTA
Twin Cities HELP
Minneapolis/St. Paul, MN
(800) 78-FACTS (toll-free MN only)

MISSOURI
Kansas City HELP
Kansas City, MO
(913) 599-9715
Web: http://hometown.aol.com/Ihaveittoo/index.html

Ozarks HELP
Springfield, MO
(417) 875-6424
E-mail: bobo3882000@yahoo.com
Web: http://www.ozarkshelp.com

St. Louis "SHEPH" HELP
St. Louis, MO
(636) 230-2288
E-mail: stl_sheph@yahoo.com

NEBRASKA
Omaha HELP
Omaha, NE
(402) 630-0780
E-mail: omahahelp@yoshi2me.com
Web: http://www.yoshi2me.com/omaha-help.html

NEW HAMPSHIRE
Seacoast HELP
Portsmouth, NH
(603) 436-7588
E-mail: herpesnh@yahoo.com
Web: http://www.herpessupport.org

NEW JERSEY
South Jersey HELP
Information Line Only—No Meetings Scheduled
(609) 748-2518
E-mail: hcir@netzero.com

NEW YORK
CNY HELP
Syracuse, NY
(315) 299–3517
E-mail: hello@cnyhelp.org

Long Island HELP
Plainview, NY
(631) 361-9338

New York HELP
Information Line Only—No Meetings Scheduled
(212) 414-7723
E-mail: help@nyhelp.org
Web: http://www.nyhelp.org

NORTH CAROLINA
Capital HELP
c/o Planned Parenthood
Raleigh, NC
(919) 833-7534
Web: http://www.pphsinc.org

Mountain HELP
Asheville, NC
(828) 216-2362
E-mail: mtnhelp@bellsouth.net
Web: http://www.mountainhelp.com

Triad HELP
c/o Guilford Co. Dept. of Public Health-
and-Planned Parenthood of Greensboro, NC
(336) 641-4699

Wayne County HELP
Goldsboro, NC
(919) 734-3563
E-mail: wayne_co_help@yahoo.com

OHIO
Cincinnati HELP
Cincinnati, OH
(513) 557-3435
E-mail: cincinnati_help@yahoo.com
Web: http://www.cincinnatihelp.org/

Cleveland HELP and HPV Support Group
(216) 323-9829
E-mail: clevelandhelp@prodigy.net

Dayton HELP
c/o Wright State University—Ellis Institute
Dayton, OH
(937) 775-4300

Ohio Support HELP
Columbus, OH
(614) 232-6446
E-mail: ohioabet@hotmail.com

OKLAHOMA
Tulsa HELP
c/o Planned Parenthood
Tulsa, OK
(918) 587-1101
E-mail: WeHELPinTulsa@yahoo.com
Web: http://www.yoshi2me.com/tulsa-help.html

OREGON
Portland Area HELP
Portland, OR
(503) 727-2640
E-mail: portlandareahelp@aol.com

PENNSYLVANIA
Philadelphia HELP
Philadelphia, PA
(610) 328-3813
E-mail: Philly437@hotmail.com

Tri State HELP
Pittsburgh, PA
(412) 341-8920
E-mail: Jbretz3452@aol.com

SOUTH CAROLINA
Columbia HELP
Columbia, SC
(803) 781-5280
E-mail: info@columbiahelp.com
Web: http://www.columbiahelp.com

Charleston HELP
Charleston, SC 29484-3242
(843) 670-0915
E-mail: admin@charlestonhelp.com
Web: http://www.yoshi2me.com/charleston-help.html

TEXAS
North Texas HELP
c/o Planned Parenthood of North Texas
Arlington, TX
(817) 276-8063 x 2241
Web: http://www.ppnt.org

Austin HELP
Austin, TX
(512) 247-5551
E-mail: austinhelp@austin.rr.com
Web: http://www.austinhelp.org

Houston HELP
Houston, TX
(866) 841-9139 x 2551 (toll-free)
E-mail: HoustonHELP@yahoo.com
Web: http://www.houstonhelp.org

VIRGINIA
Richmond HELP
c/o Fan Free Clinic
Richmond, VA
(804) 358-6343

Rappahannock HELP
Fredericksburg, VA
(540) 371-0934
E-mail: rappahannockhelp@aol.com

WEST VIRGINIA
Northcentral West Virginia HELP
c/o West Virginia University
Morgantown, WV
(304) 293-6584
E-mail: pkovac@hsc.wvu.edu
Web: http://www.hsc.wvu.edu

CANADA
Alberta
Calgary HELP
Calgary, AB
(403) 228-7400

British Columbia
Vancouver HELP
Vancouver, BC
(604) 515-5500
Web: http://groups.yahoo.com/group/vancouverhelp/

Manitoba
Winnipeg HELP
Winnipeg, MB
(204) 940-2200

Ontario
Toronto HELP
c/o The Phoenix Association
Toronto, ON
(416) 449-0876
E-mail: phoenix_association@hotmail.com
E-mail: phoenix_association@hotmail.com
Web: http://www.torontoherpes.com

Quebec
Montreal HELP
St. Laurent, QC
(514) 855-8995
E-mail: ruban-en-route@qc.aira.com
Web: http://www.rubanenroute.org/herpes.php

AUSTRALIA
Sydney HELP
c/o Sydney Sexual Health Centre
Sydney, NSW—Australia
61 2 382-7440
Web: http://www.sydneysexualhealthcentre.com.au

Appendix B

Publications

The helper, a quarterly newsletter published by the nonprofit American Social Health Association, provides updates on herpes research and helpful information about coping with genital herpes.
Cost: $25 for a one-year subscription.
Ordering: 1-919-361-8488 or write to ASHA, Department T, PO Box 13827, Research Triangle Park, NC 27709. Online ordering at https://www.ashastd.org/publications/publications_ind.cfm

Managing Herpes: How to Live and Love with a Chronic STD, 3rd Edition, ASHA, Research Triangle Park, NC. This award-winning book by Charles Ebel of the American Social Health Association and Anna Wald of the University of Washington is a thorough and informative guide to the medical and emotional aspects of herpes.
Cost: $26.95
Ordering: 1-919-361-8488 or write to ASHA, Department T, PO Box 13827, Research Triangle Park, NC 27709. Online ordering at https://www.ashastd.org/publications/publications_ind.cfm

Understanding Herpes, ASHA, Research Triangle Park, NC. This 16-page pamphlet intended for the person who has recently acquired genital herpes contains information about symptoms, treatment, and spread of the infection and how to deal with the social and psychological pressures.

It comes with two brochures, *Telling Your Partner* and
When Your Partner Has Herpes.

Cost: $7.

Ordering: 1-919-361-8488 or write to ASHA, Department T,
PO Box 13827, Research Triangle Park, NC 27709.
Online ordering at https://www.ashastd.org/publications/
publications_ind.cfm

Appendix C

The Internet

The network of computers known as the Internet is a remarkable source of information concerning herpes. The information is similar to that gained in conversations with strangers at informal parties: some comes from knowledgeable people, some represents the opinions of those who are uninformed, and some is calculated to best serve the interests of the speaker, not necessarily the listener. Be very cautious about using this medium; try to determine who has created a specific Web site (Internet address) and why. These sites can be expensive to set up and maintain, so ask yourself why someone is doing it. With regard to herpes, the answer generally falls into one of four categories: (1) they have something to sell you and hope that, if they offer you information about a condition, you will decide that their product (drug, vaccine, herbal remedy, or dating service) would be useful in managing that condition (be wary of Web sites that offer unproved remedies); (2) they are involved in public health issues and provide the site in order to help teach the public about herpes; (3) they are engaged in health research and seek to educate you and potentially enlist your help in ongoing clinical research; (4) they have been personally affected by herpes simplex virus infection and want to inform the public regarding this very common condition. Some Web sites are intended primarily for the general public, while others are designed for health care professionals. Some provide links to a wide variety of related sites, which can be useful in helping you locate the best and most frequently visited ones. The following is a limited list of Web sites with brief comments regarding what you might find there. This is not an endorsement of any of the sites but is intended to serve as a starting place for an exploration of this source of extensive information. As with so many other aspects of herpes, remember the Latin warning *caveat emptor*—let the buyer beware!

Address: http://www.ashastd.org/herpes/herpes_overview.cfm
Web site: National Herpes Resource Center
Comments: An outstanding website provided by the American Social Health Association. This site provides up to date information regarding genital herpes and information about the national herpes hotline and a chat room.

Address: http://www.herpesdiagnosis.com/
Web site: Herpes Diagnosis
Comments: This website was designed by Drs. Lawrence Corey, Rhoda Ashley Morrow, and Gray Davis, all experts in genital herpes. The site provides accurate information about herpes diagnosis and treatment. The site is somewhat oriented to healthcare professionals.

Address: http://www.ihmf.org/
Web site: International Herpesvirus Management Forum
Comments: The International Herpes Management Forum was established in 1993 to improve the awareness and understanding of herpesviruses, and the counseling and management of people with these infections. The site is somewhat oriented towards health professionals but contains up-to-date scientific information regarding herpes virus infections.

Address: http://www.westoverheights.com/index.html
Web site: Westover Heights Clinic
Comments: A site maintained by Terri Warren, RN, ANP, containing patient oriented information including a national

list of healthcare providers who are felt to be providers of good herpes care.

Address: http://www.herpes-foundation.org/
Web site: American Herpes Foundation
Comments: A quality site maintained by the American Herpes Foundation, a not-for-profit organization dedicated to providing information and clinical education about genital herpes.

Address: http://www.cdc.gov/std/Herpes/STDFact-Herpes.htm
Web site: Genital Herpes—CDC Fact Sheet
Comments: A fact sheet developed by the U.S. Centers for Disease Control and Prevention.

Address: http://www.niaid.nih.gov/factsheets/stdherp.htm
Web site: Genital Herpes Fact Sheet
Comments: A fact sheet developed by the U.S. National Institute of Allergy and Infectious Disease that provides up to date information about the diagnosis and treatment of genital herpes and ongoing research for the treatment and control of genital herpes.

Address: http://my.webmd.com/medical_information/condition_centers/genital_herpes/default.htm
Web site: Genital Herpes Health Center
Comments: A site by Web MD that provides basic information on herpes and maintains an outstanding message board moderated by Terri Warren RN, APN, a nationally recognized researcher and expert on genital herpes and nurse practitioner at Westover Heights Clinic in Portland, Oregon.

Address: http://www.goaskalice.Columbia.edu/Cat7.html
Web site: Go Ask Alice site

Comments: A site developed by Columbia University's Health Education Service, it allows readers to ask questions about sexual health, general health, and relationship topics. Readers can also browse past questions and answers regarding herpes and other related topics.

Address: http://www.herpesdiagnosis.com/
Web site: Herpes Diagnosis
Comments: This site provides up-to-date information about the tests that can be used to diagnosis herpes—not all available tests are accurate and this site can help the patient sort out the complexities of available blood tests.

Address: http://www.tstd.org/
Web site: tSTD.org
Comments: tSTD is a new anonymous testing service that offers Focus Technologies' HerpeSelect® 1 and 2 ELISA IgG tests to detect herpes simplex virus types 1 and 2. This test is one of the few accurate commercially available herpes blood tests.

Address: http://www.herpeshelp.com/
Web site: HerpesHelp.com
Comments: A site sponsored by GlaxoSmithKline, the maker of valacyclovir (Valtrex®). This site has herpes facts and treatment options for genital herpes and information of prevention of the spread of genital herpes.

Address: http://www.healthandhope.com/index.jsp?checked=y
Web site: H.O.P.E. (Herpes Outreach Patient Education)
A web site by Novartis Pharmaceuticals, the makers of the antiviral drug famciclovir (Famvir®), that contains information about living with and dealing with genital herpes.

Address: http://www.mpwh.net/
Web site: Antopia Network
Comments: The site provides a dating service for people with herpes as well as links to local social organizations for people with herpes.

Glossary

Acyclovir   An antiviral drug used in the treatment of herpes simplex virus infections.

Adjuvant   A chemical agent used to increase the potency of a vaccine.

Anterograde transport   Material (virus) within a nerve fiber moving from the cell body (nucleus) out to the periphery of the nerve.

Antibodies   Complex proteins made by the body's immune system, found in the blood and other bodily fluids and involved in fighting disease-causing microbes.

Asymptomatic recurrences   Silent outbreaks in which the only evidence of the recurrence is the presence of the virus on skin or mucous membranes (also referred to as subclinical or unrecognized shedding).

Attenuate   To weaken a microbe so that it can be used as a vaccine.

Cesarean section   A surgical procedure that involves making an incision in the abdomen and uterus and delivering the baby through the incision.

Chancres   Large and sometimes painful ulcers which can be mistaken for herpes sores but are usually caused by syphilis.

Crust   A thin scab covering a sore.

Cutaneous   Relating to the skin.

Cytokines   Non-antibody proteins involved in host defense against disease-causing microbes.

Deoxyribonucleic acid (DNA)   A large complex chemical molecule that contains the genetic code for organisms (from viruses to human beings) and serves as a blueprint for the organism's reproduction.

Discordant couples   Partners in a sexual relationship in which one person (the source partner) has genital herpes and the other (the exposed partner) does not, being therefore at risk of becoming infected.

Disseminated infection   A widespread herpes simplex virus infection that moves from the skin to the bloodstream and may involve internal organs.

Dysuria   Difficult or painful urination.

Encephalitis   An infection of the central nervous system (brain).

Envelope   The outermost membrane-like structure of a virus made of carbohydrates, lipids, and proteins.

Epidemiology   Scientific discipline that studies the occurrence of disease in populations.

Erythema   Abnormal redness of the skin.

False prodrome   A situation in which the telltale prodromal symptoms that can predict a coming outbreak of herpes are noted but the individual fails to develop the predicted genital lesions.

Famciclovir   A new antiviral drug used in treating herpes simplex virus infections.

First episode   The first development of recognizable signs and symptoms of genital herpes.

Ganglion   (plural, **ganglia**) A discrete collection or mass of nerve cells which send forth nerve fibers. Herpes simplex virus moves from the skin through the nerve fibers to the nerve cells in ganglia, where the latent infection is harbored.

Herpes encephalitis   An uncommon illness in which the brain becomes infected with herpes simplex virus.

Herpes gingivostomatitis   A painful infection of the mouth generally caused by herpes simplex virus type 1 and common in childhood.

Herpes keratitis   A relatively common infection of the eye caused by herpes simplex virus, which can be serious and may lead to blindness.

Herpes pharyngitis   Sore throat caused by herpes simplex virus infection of the tonsils and/or lining of the throat.

Humoral immunity   Antibodies and other microbe-fighting factors found in bodily fluids.

Immunocompromised host   An individual whose immune system is diminished, impaired, or absent.

Immunogenicity   The ability of a vaccine to induce specific immune responses against a disease-causing microbe; can be characterized by the magnitude and duration of specific immune responses as well as by type of response, i.e., humoral or cellular.

Immunopotentiation   Enhancement of the immune response; usually refers to the addition of adjuvants to a vaccine so as to increase immunogenicity.

Inactivated vaccines   Consist of whole killed microbes that are incapable of causing disease; good at inducing the immune system to make antibodies against the organism but less effective in inducing cellular immune responses.

Incubation period   The time between a person's exposure to a contagious disease-causing microbe and the development of signs and symptoms of the illness.

Intraneural   Inside a nerve.

Intrapartum infection   Spread of infection from the mother to the baby during the labor and delivery period.

Intrauterine infection   Spread of infection from the mother to the fetus within the uterus; may occur anytime during the pregnancy.

Latency or latent infection   An inactive state, like hibernation, in which herpes simplex virus persists in nerve cells without causing disease.

Live-attenuated vaccines Contain whole microbes that have been weakened so they cannot cause disease, but, because they can still multiply (replicate), they cause the body to produce both antibody and cellular immune responses against the disease-causing microbe.

Live-vectored vaccines Specially engineered vaccines that consist of a live-attenuated microbe (the vector) in which a small piece of genetic information from a different disease-causing microbe has been inserted. A person receiving such a vaccine makes immune responses not only to the vector but also to the extra bit of the disease-causing microbe. This is a way to piggyback parts of dangerous microbes so that they can be safely given to humans.

Microbe A tiny microorganism; usually refers to disease-causing bacteria or viruses; a germ.

Mucosal cells Moist cells such as those found inside the mouth or genital tract.

Neonatal herpes A potentially life-threatening herpes simplex virus infection of the newborn infant.

Neonate An infant in the first month of life.

Nonprimary first episode genital herpes Generally caused by the type 2 virus and occurring in a person who has previously had a nongenital type 1 virus infection such as herpes labialis (fever blisters/cold sores). The prior nongenital infection may have been unrecognized and only detected by blood tests that measure antibody against the type 1 virus.

Nucleic acid-based vaccines Sometimes referred to as naked DNA vaccines and still very experimental. Scientists have shown that immunization with small pieces of DNA or RNA from a disease-causing microbe can protect animals from disease caused by the microbe.

Penciclovir A new antiviral drug that is used in the treatment of herpes labialis (fever blisters).

Placebo effect   A phenomenon whereby people perceive improvement in a medical condition when they are receiving a treatment known to be ineffective, such as a sugar pill.

Polymerase chain reaction (PCR)   A newly developed and highly sensitive method to detect DNA; the basis of new diagnostic tests for herpes simplex virus infections.

Prodrome   Premonitory symptoms that occur one to two days before the development of recurrent herpes lesions.

Reactivation   The reawakening of a latent infection.

Reactogenicity   The tendency of a vaccine to cause undesirable reactions such as pain at the site of injection, headache, muscle ache, or fever.

Recurrences or recurrent infections   The outbreaks of herpes sores that are experienced after a person has recovered from a first episode of disease.

Replication-impaired viral vaccine   Consists of viruses that have been genetically engineered so that they can only undergo a single round of replication but not produce more virus. Such impaired viruses induce broad immune responses but do not multiply enough to cause disease.

Self-limited   Descriptive of an illness or disease that eventually improves without treatment.

Seroprevalence   An estimate of how many people in any population have antibodies to the microbe of interest, allowing scientists to determine how many people have been infected with a particular disease-causing microbe.

Serum   The liquid portion of blood remaining after blood clots.

Sign   An objective finding made by a doctor; an example would be a swollen lymph gland.

Subclinical   An infection which causes no signs or symptoms readily ascribed to the infection.

Subclinical shedding   Silent recurrences or outbreaks in which the only evidence of the recurrence is the presence of the virus on skin or mucous membranes (also referred to as asymptomatic or unrecognized shedding).

Subunit vaccines   Contain small pieces or subunits of the microbe, usually protein components of the outer structure of the organism.

Symptom   A subjective finding, associated with an illness, which is reported by a patient to a doctor; an example would be tenderness in a swollen lymph gland.

True primary infection   The first time a person is infected with either type of herpes simplex virus; must be defined by blood tests collected when a person is first thought to be infected.

Ulcers   Shallow erosions in the skin.

Unrecognized shedding   Silent recurrences or outbreaks in which the only evidence of the recurrence is the presence of the virus on skin or mucous membranes (also referred to as asymptomatic recurrences or subclinical shedding).

Urethra   The canal or tube that allows urine to pass from the bladder to the outside of the body.

Urethritis   Inflammation of the urethra, usually manifested by a clear discharge or drip and/or dysuria.

Valacyclovir   A new antiviral drug used in treating herpes simplex virus infections.

Vesicles   Small blister-like lesions on the skin or mucous membranes; may contain clear or yellow fluid.

Virion   An elementary virus particle.

Virulent   Describes a microbe's ability to cause severe disease.

Virus   A tiny microbe capable of passing through fine filters and incapable of reproduction outside a living cell.

Index

Understanding Health and Sickness Series
Miriam Bloom, Ph.D., General Editor

Also in this series

Addiction • Alzheimer's Disease • Anemia • Asthma • Breast Cancer
Genetics • Cancer Therapies • Child Sexual Abuse • Childhood
Obesity • Chronic Pain • Colon Cancer • Cosmetic Laser Surgery •
Crohn Disease and Ulcerative Colitis • Cystic Fibrosis • Dental
Health • Depression • Hepatitis • Mental Retardation • Migraine and
Other Headaches • Multiple Sclerosis • Panic and Other Anxiety
Disorders • Sickle Cell Disease • Stuttering

DATE DUE

MAY 1 4 2009			

HIGHSMITH 45231